SUGAR DETOX

Publications International, Ltd.

Microwave Cooking: Microwave ovens vary in wattage. Use the cooking times as guidelines and check for doneness before adding more time.

WHAT EXACTLY ARE CARBOHYDRATES?

You know that carbohydrates are sugars and starches found in fruits, vegetables and grains. While that's true, it's hardly the whole picture, since junk food like soda pop, pizza, potato chips and cupcakes are also packed with carbs. Clearly, some carbohydrate-rich foods are healthier than others. Most of the carbohydrates in your diet should come from healthy sources, such as fruits, vegetables and whole grains.

Potatoes and pinto beans. Carrots and cauliflower. Rye bread and rock candy. Juice and soda pop. These foods have one thing in common: They're all sources of carbohydrates. They come in all shapes and sizes. They're found in fruits, vegetables, grains, beans, dairy products and just about everything other than meat, fish or fat. Broadly speaking, carbohydrates fall into three categories:

Sugars

The word "sugar" may make you think of the white granules you spoon into coffee or add to baked goods, but the sweet stuff comes in many varieties. Sugars are the simplest form of carbohydrates and include sucrose (found in table sugar and some fruits and vegetables), fructose (found in fruit and honey) and lactose (found in milk), among others.

Starches

Although they consist of sugar units, the complex structure of starches makes them a distinct type of carbohydrate. The large size of starch molecules also sets them apart from sugars; they're too big for taste bud receptors on the tongue, which is why starches usually don't taste sweet. Starchy foods include potatoes, bread, pasta and rice.

It is important to go with the (whole) grain. White flour is produced by grinding wheat to remove the sturdy outer layers of the grain, known as the bran and germ. Unfortunately, this refining process not only strips away the bran and germ, but also removes lots of fiber, vitamins (especially vitamins B and E) and minerals, too. The same thing happens when rice is processed to make it pearly white.

Whole grain breads, pasta and rice are made with the entire grain, and have a bolder taste and chewier texture than most of their paler cousins. Over time, you may find that white bread and other refined grains taste bland. Beware of imitators: Some commercial bakeries sell "wheat" bread that is simply white bread that has been dyed brown. Pasta makers sometimes dye pasta brown, too, to make it appear healthier. Look for the words "whole grain" or "whole wheat" on packages.

Your gut calls it "indigestible." Fiber is made up of an intricate array of sugar molecules like starch, but these sugar molecules aren't absorbed into the bloodstream because the body lacks enzymes to break them down. Even though fiber isn't technically a nutrient, it does plenty of good.

Dietary fiber is a key component to the success in any diet. Fiber has been proven effective in disease prevention, weight loss and blood sugar control. It's naturally present in plants and therefore is a major nutritional component of fruits, vegetables, beans, nuts, seeds and whole grains. While many processed food products do have some added fiber, the best sources are natural, unrefined foods.

Dietary fiber slows down the process of digestion, which gives the brain time to receive the message that the stomach is full. Also, fiber slows down the breakdown of food to glucose, moderating the blood glucose rise that occurs after any meal.

There are two types of dietary fiber, insoluble and soluble fiber, and both play an important role in weight loss. Insoluble fiber increases the bulk in the stomach, while soluble fiber slows down the digestive processes. As a result, you feel fuller from a smaller amount of food for an extended period of time.

Most of the fiber we consume is insoluble fiber. This type of fiber increases the weight and size of your stool, which allows regular bowel movements to occur, preventing constipation and aiding in digestive health. If you want to increase the fiber to your diet, just be cautious not to add too much too quickly, or to increase the amount of fiber in your diet without increasing your water intake. A drastic increase of fiber in the diet can cause abdominal discomfort, gas and constipation.

Soluble fiber—commonly found in beans, oats, and the peels of apples—absorbs water, providing a feeling of fullness as you eat, which helps you avoid overeating. It also slows down the digestive processes, helping to delay the blood glucose response after a meal.

Soluble fiber plays an important role in heart health, too. When bound to water, soluble fiber forms a gel-like substance in the digestive tract that absorbs cholesterol and carries it out of the body. This reduces blood cholesterol levels, helping to reduce the risk of heart disease.

PORTION DISTORTION

Regardless of what you're eating, one of the most important things that you should pay attention to is portion size. Learning to recognize all of the ingredients in a dish and the recommended serving sizes are fundamental tools to the success of any healthy lifestyle. Use the serving size listed on the Nutrition Facts panel on any packaged food or the nutrition information listed with the recipes in this book as a guide. The nutrition information listed with each recipe is based on a single serving and does not include garnishes or optional ingredients; when a range is given for an ingredient, the nutritional analysis reflects the lesser amount. Please consult a registered dietitian or health care provider who can offer nutrition advice, tips and meal plans that are all specific to your lifestyle.

FOODS TO ENJOY

All Meat, Seafood, Nuts, Seeds, Spices, Eggs and Butter

Whole Grains: brown rice, quinoa, millet, barley, buckwheat, farro, oats, wild rice

Low-Carb Vegetables: bok choy, celery, spinach, asparagus, radishes, avocado, zucchini, mushrooms, tomatoes, olives, eggplant, bell pepper, cauliflower, cabbage, cucumber

Low-Carb Fruits: berries, peaches, kiwi, grapefruit, honeydew, coconut, apple, lime, apricot, pear, plum, nectarines, oranges, cantaloupe

Legumes and Beans: lentils, chickpeas, kidney beans, navy beans, black beans

Beverages: tea, water, unsweetened almond/nut milks

Condiments: apple cider vinegar, red wine vinegar, olive oil, coconut oil, sesame oil

FOODS TO LIMIT

Dairy, high-carb fruits and vegetables

FOODS TO AVOID

Artificial sweeteners and dried fruit

Sugar: raw sugar, brown sugar, white sugar, coconut sugar, confectioner's sugar, agave nectar, maple syrup, molasses, corn syrup, honey

Refined Flours: white bread, pretzels, bagels, cookies, cakes, brownies

Beverages: alcohol, juice, soda, sweetened tea

Condiments: check all labels for added sugar

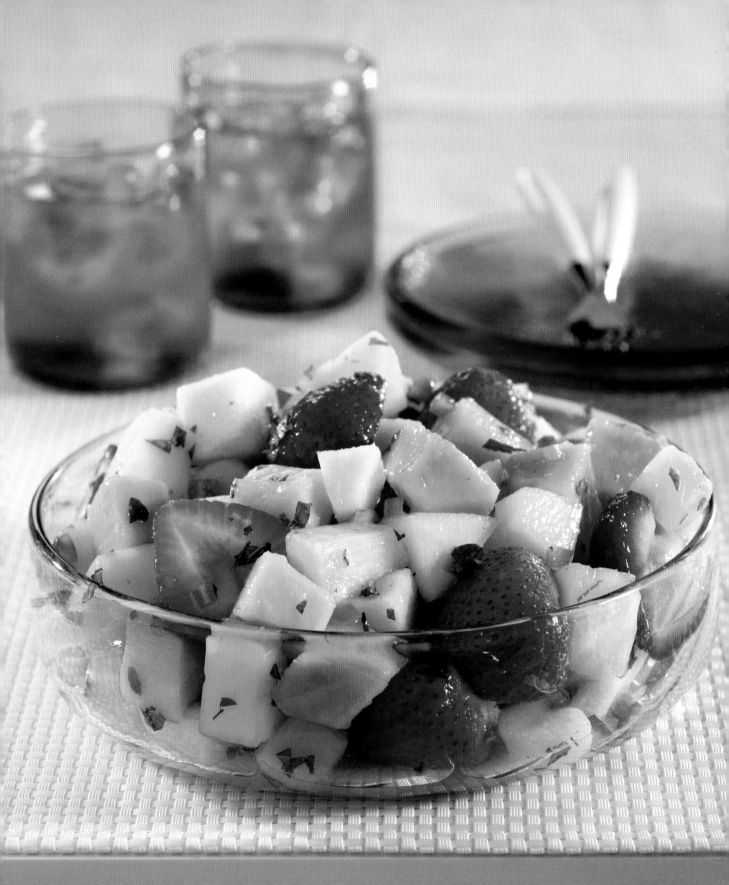

BREAKFAST

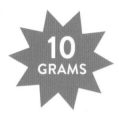

10 GRAMS

HOT AND SPICY FRUIT SALAD

makes 12 servings

⅓ cup fresh orange juice

3 tablespoons lime juice

3 tablespoons minced fresh mint, basil or cilantro, plus additional for garnish

2 jalapeño peppers,* seeded, minced

½ small honeydew melon, cut into cubes

½ ripe large papaya, peeled, seeded, cubed

1 cup fresh strawberries, stemmed, halved

1 can (8 ounces) pineapple chunks, drained

*Jalapeño peppers can sting and irritate the skin, so wear rubber gloves when handling peppers and do not touch your eyes.

1. Blend orange juice, lime juice, 3 tablespoons mint and jalapeño peppers in small bowl.

2. Combine melon, papaya, strawberries and pineapple in large bowl. Pour orange juice mixture over fruit; toss gently until well blended.

3. Serve immediately or cover and refrigerate up to 3 hours. Garnish with additional fresh mint, if desired.

nutritionals

Serving Size: *½ cup*, Calories: *50*, Total Fat: *0g*, Saturated Fat: *0g*, Cholesterol: *0mg*, Sodium: *10mg*, Carbohydrate: *12g*, Dietary Fiber: *1g*, Sugar: *10g*, Protein: *1g*

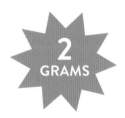

2 GRAMS

FETA BRUNCH BAKE

makes 4 servings

1   medium red bell pepper

2   bags (10 ounces each) fresh spinach, stemmed

6   eggs

1½ cups (6 ounces) crumbled feta cheese

⅓   cup chopped onion

2   tablespoons chopped fresh parsley

¼   teaspoon dried dill weed

     Dash black pepper

1. Preheat broiler. Place bell pepper on foil-lined broiler pan. Broil 4 inches from heat source 15 to 20 minutes or until blackened on all sides, turning every 5 minutes with tongs. Place in paper bag; close bag and set aside to cool 15 to 20 minutes. Remove core; cut bell pepper in half and rub off skin. Rinse under cold water. Cut into ½-inch pieces.

2. Fill medium saucepan half full with water; bring to a boil over high heat. Add spinach; return to a boil. Boil 2 to 3 minutes or until wilted. Drain spinach; immediately plunge spinach into medium bowl of cold water. Drain; let stand until cool enough to handle. Squeeze spinach to remove excess water; finely chop.

3. Preheat oven to 400°F. Spray 1-quart baking dish with nonstick cooking spray.

4. Beat eggs in large bowl with electric mixer at medium speed until foamy. Stir in roasted pepper, spinach, cheese, onion, parsley, dill weed and black pepper. Pour into prepared baking dish.

5. Bake 20 minutes or until set. Let stand 5 minutes before serving. Cut evenly into four squares to serve.

nutritionals

Serving Size: *1 square*, Calories: *280*, Total Fat: *18g*, Saturated Fat: *9g*, Cholesterol: *300mg*, Sodium: *750mg*, Carbohydrate: *10g*, Dietary Fiber: *4g*, Sugar: *2g*, Protein: *21g*

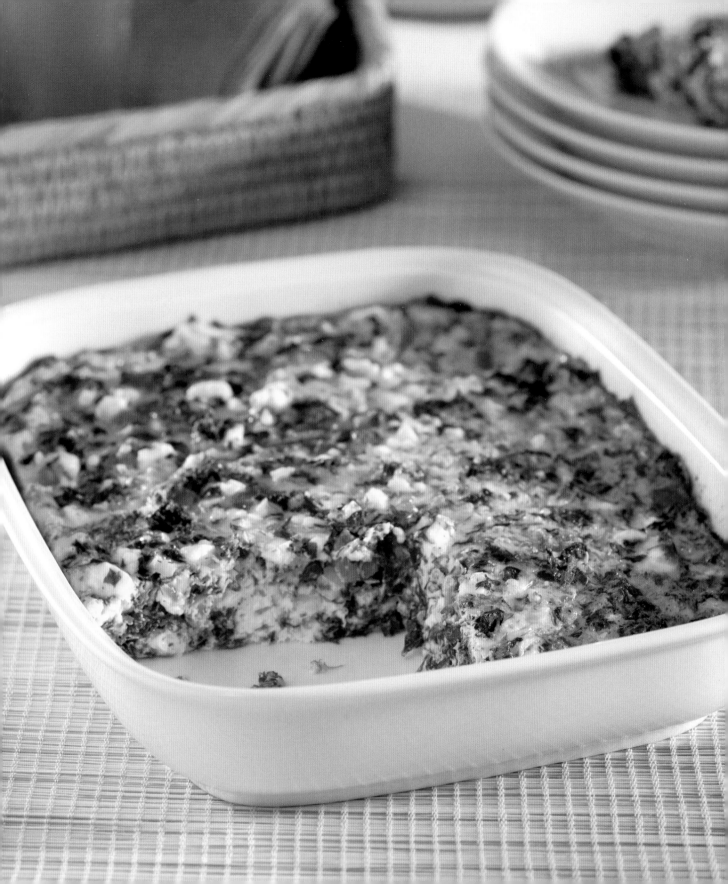

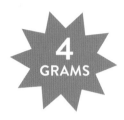

4 GRAMS

MICROWAVED OATS CEREAL

makes 2 servings

1¾ cups water

⅓ cup old-fashioned oats

⅓ cup oat bran

¼ teaspoon ground cinnamon

⅛ teaspoon salt

½ cup fresh blueberries

MICROWAVE DIRECTIONS

1. Combine water, oats, oat bran, cinnamon and salt in large microwavable bowl (cereal expands rapidly when it cooks). Cover with vented plastic wrap.

2. Microwave on HIGH 6 minutes or until thickened. Stir well. Let stand 2 minutes before serving. Top evenly with blueberries.

SERVING SUGGESTION: You may also add fresh strawberries and/or nuts to this quick morning meal.

nutritionals

Serving Size: *1 cup*, Calories: *110*, Total Fat: *2g*, Saturated Fat: *0g*, Cholesterol: *0mg*, Sodium: *150mg*, Carbohydrate: *25g*, Dietary Fiber: *5g*, Sugar: *4g*, Protein: *5g*

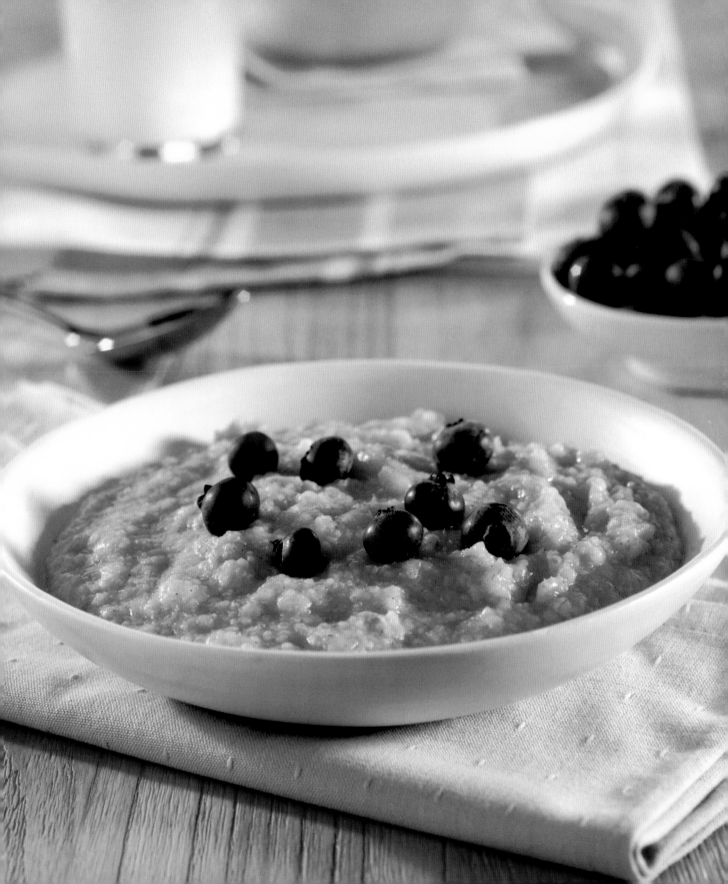

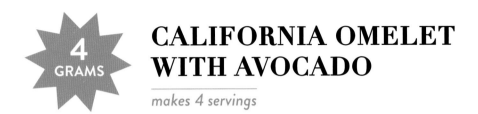

4 GRAMS

CALIFORNIA OMELET WITH AVOCADO

makes 4 servings

6 ounces plum tomato, chopped (about 1½ tomatoes)

2 to 4 tablespoons chopped fresh cilantro

¼ teaspoon salt

8 eggs

¼ cup milk

1 ripe medium avocado, diced

1 small cucumber, chopped

1 lemon, quartered

1. Preheat oven to 200°F. Combine tomatoes, cilantro and salt in small bowl; set aside.

2. Whisk eggs and milk in medium bowl until blended. Heat small nonstick skillet over medium heat. Pour half of egg mixture into skillet; cook 2 minutes or until eggs begin to set. Lift edge of omelet to allow uncooked portion to flow underneath. Cook 3 minutes or until set.

3. Spoon half of tomato mixture over half of omelet. Loosen omelet with spatula and fold in half. Slide omelet onto serving plates and keep warm in oven. Repeat steps for second omelet with remaining half of egg mixture. Serve with avocado, cucumber and lemon.

nutritionals

Serving Size: *½ omelet*, Calories: *250*, Total Fat: *17g*, Saturated Fat: *5g*, Cholesterol: *375mg*, Sodium: *300mg*, Carbohydrate: *11g*, Dietary Fiber: *5g*, Sugar: *4g*, Protein: *15g*

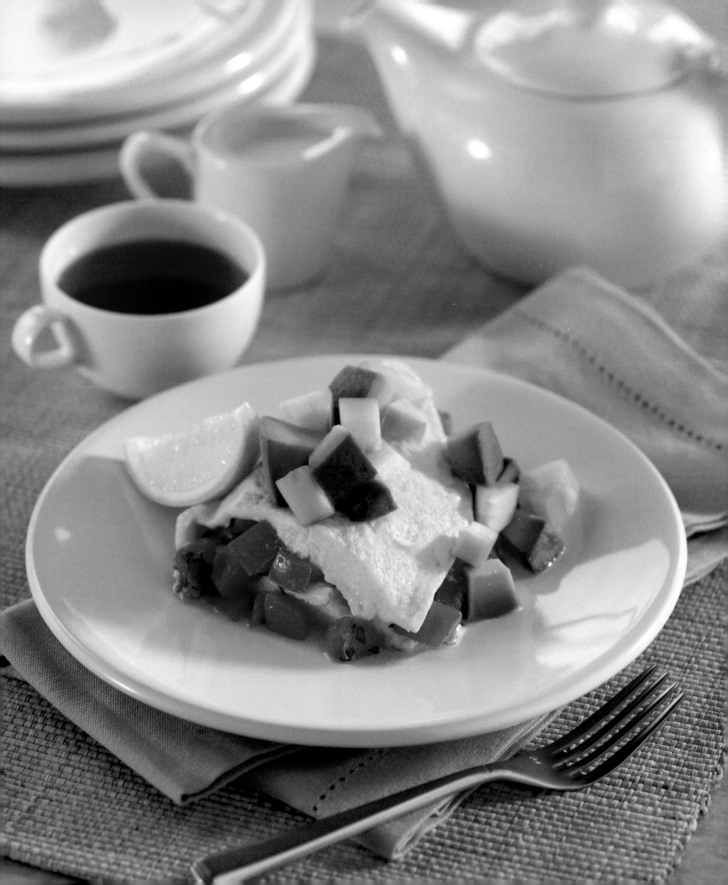

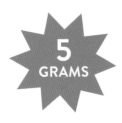

5 GRAMS

WHOA BREAKFAST

makes 6 servings

3 cups water

2 cups chopped peeled apples

1½ cups steel-cut or old-fashioned oats

¼ cup sliced almonds

½ teaspoon ground cinnamon, plus additional for garnish

Sliced apples (optional)

SLOW COOKER DIRECTIONS

Combine water, chopped apples, oats, almonds and ½ teaspoon cinnamon in slow cooker. Cover; cook on LOW 8 hours. Garnish each serving with apple slices and additional cinnamon.

nutritionals

Serving Size: *about ½ cup*, Calories: *190*, Total Fat: *5g*, Saturated Fat: *1g*, Cholesterol: *0mg*, Sodium: *0mg*, Carbohydrate: *33g*, Dietary Fiber: *5g*, Sugar: *5g*, Protein: *6g*

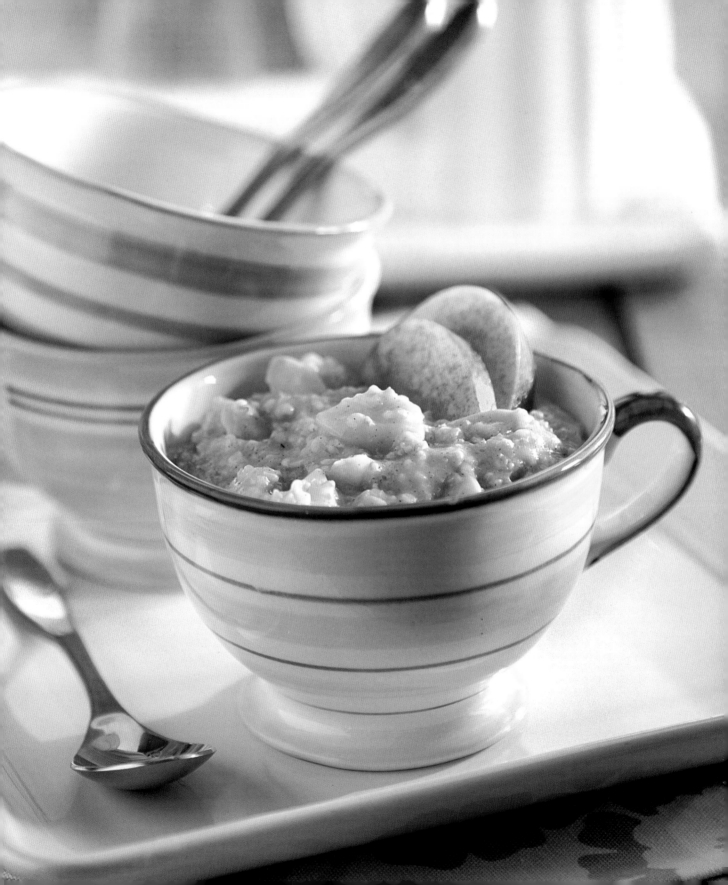

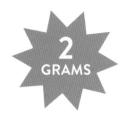

2 GRAMS

INDIVIDUAL SPINACH & BACON QUICHES

makes 12 servings

3 slices bacon

½ small onion, diced

1 package (10 ounces) frozen chopped spinach, thawed and squeezed dry

½ teaspoon black pepper

⅛ teaspoon ground nutmeg

Pinch salt

1 container (15 ounces) whole-milk ricotta cheese

2 cups (8 ounces) shredded mozzarella cheese

1 cup grated Parmesan cheese

3 eggs, lightly beaten

1. Preheat oven to 350°F. Spray 12 standard (2½-inch) muffin cups with nonstick cooking spray.

2. Cook bacon in large skillet over medium-high heat until crisp. Drain on paper towel-lined plate. Reserve drippings in skillet. Crumble bacon.

3. Add onion to skillet; cook and stir 5 minutes or until tender. Add spinach, pepper, nutmeg and salt; cook and stir over medium heat 3 minutes or until liquid is evaporated. Remove from heat. Stir in crumbled bacon; set aside to cool.

4. Combine cheeses in large bowl. Add eggs; stir until well blended. Add cooled spinach mixture; mix well. Spoon evenly into prepared muffin cups.

5. Bake 40 minutes or until set. Let stand 10 minutes. Run thin knife around edges to remove from pan. Serve immediately.

nutritionals

Serving Size: *1 quiche*, Calories: *180*, Total Fat: *12g*, Saturated Fat: *7g*, Cholesterol: *75mg*, Sodium: *430mg*, Carbohydrate: *4g*, Dietary Fiber: *1g*, Sugar: *2g*, Protein: *16g*

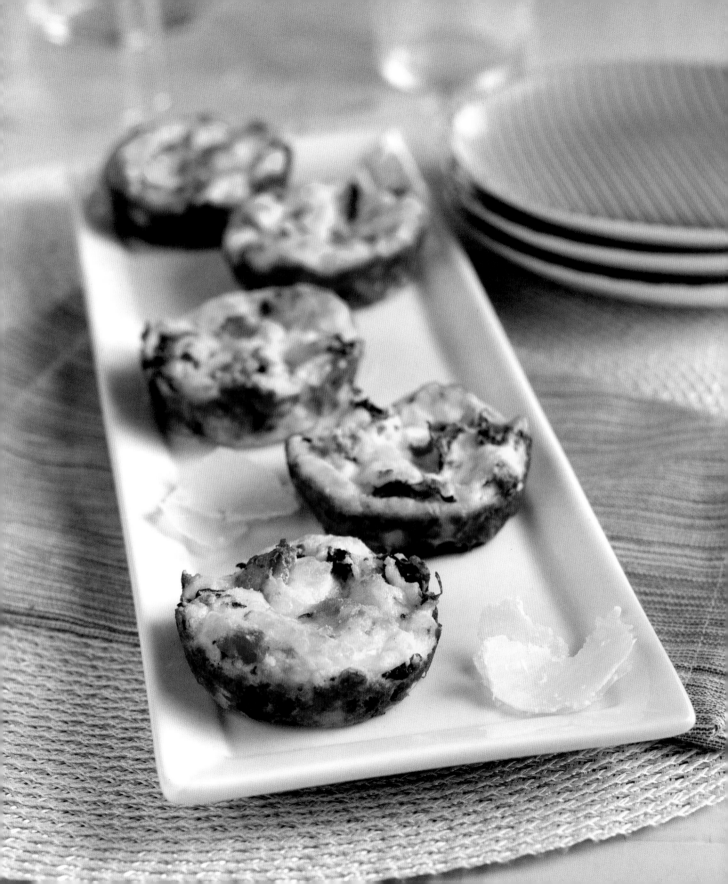

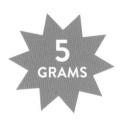

5 GRAMS

PEA AND SPINACH FRITTATA

makes 4 servings

1 cup chopped onion

¼ cup water

1 cup frozen peas

1 cup fresh spinach

6 egg whites

2 eggs

½ cup cooked brown rice

¼ cup milk

2 tablespoons grated Romano
   or Parmesan cheese, plus
   additional for garnish

1 tablespoon chopped fresh
   mint *or* 1 teaspoon dried
   mint, crushed

¼ teaspoon black pepper

⅛ teaspoon salt

1. Spray large skillet with nonstick cooking spray. Combine onion and water in skillet; bring to a boil over high heat. Reduce heat to medium. Cover; cook 2 to 3 minutes or until onion is tender. Stir in peas; cook until heated through. Drain. Add spinach; cook and stir 1 minute or until spinach just begins to wilt.

2. Combine egg whites, eggs, rice, milk, 2 tablespoons Romano cheese, mint, pepper and salt in medium bowl. Add egg mixture to skillet. Cook, without stirring, 2 minutes or until eggs begin to set. Run large spoon around edge of skillet, lifting eggs for even cooking. Remove skillet from heat when eggs are almost set but surface is still moist.

3. Cover; let stand 3 to 4 minutes or until surface is set. Sprinkle with additional Romano cheese, if desired. Cut into four wedges to serve.

---

nutritionals

Serving Size: *1 wedge*, Calories: *160*, Total Fat: *4g*, Saturated Fat: *2g*, Cholesterol: *95mg*, Sodium: *300mg*, Carbohydrate: *16g*, Dietary Fiber: *3g*, Sugar: *5g*, Protein: *13g*

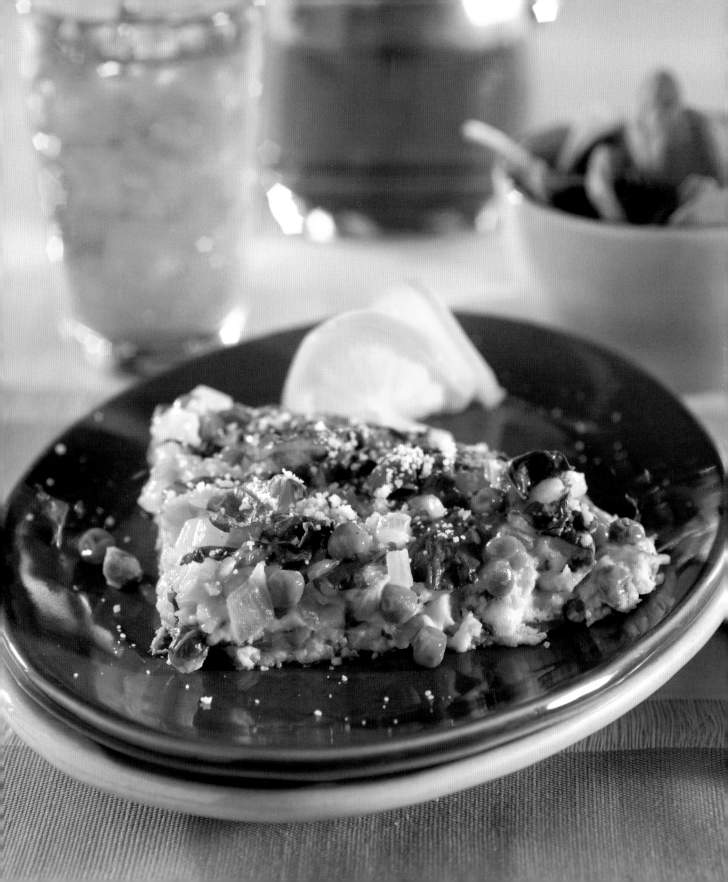

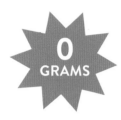

0 GRAMS

LEMON AND BASIL TEA

makes 16 servings

¾ cup plus 2 tablespoons loose English breakfast tea leaves

2 tablespoons lemon peel

2 tablespoons fresh basil

16 cups water

Lemon wedges (optional)

Combine tea leaves, lemon peel and basil in coffee filter; place in top of coffee maker. Pour water into coffee maker; turn on to brew tea. Pour into mugs. Serve with lemon wedges.

nutritionals

Serving Size: *about ½ cup*, Calories: *0*, Total Fat: *0g*, Saturated Fat: *0g*, Cholesterol: *0mg*, Sodium: *0mg*, Carbohydrate: *0g*, Dietary Fiber: *0g*, Sugar: *0g*, Protein: *0g*

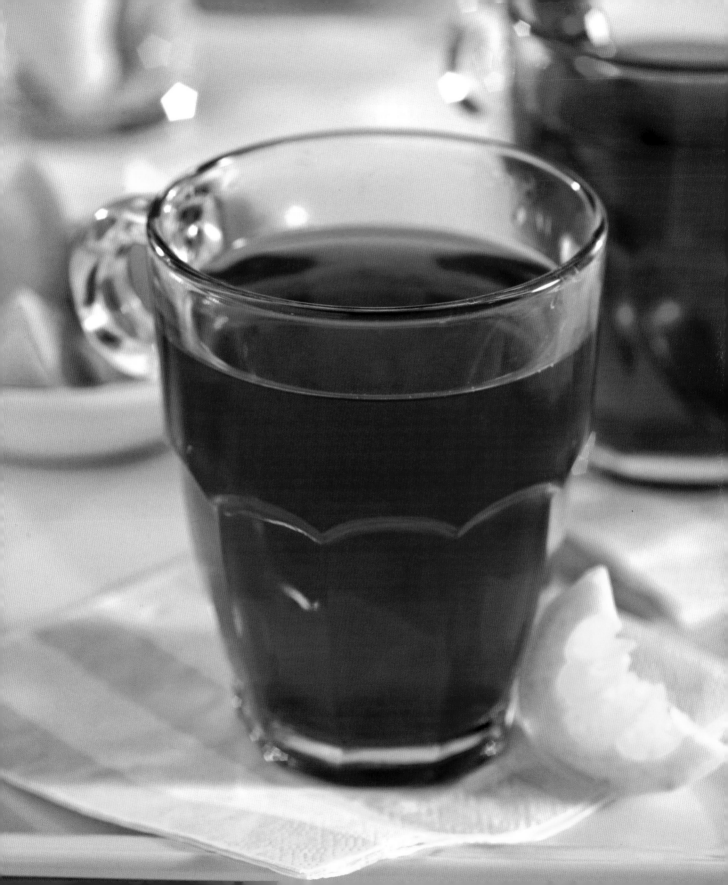

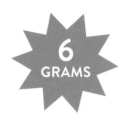

6 GRAMS

CRUSTLESS HAM & SPINACH TART

makes 6 servings

1   teaspoon olive oil

1   cup finely chopped onion

2   cloves garlic, minced

1   package (10 ounces) frozen chopped spinach, thawed and squeezed dry

3   slices deli ham, cut into strips (3 ounces total)

1   cup milk

3   eggs

¼   cup plus 2 tablespoons grated Parmesan cheese, divided

1   tablespoon minced fresh basil *or* 2 teaspoons dried basil

½   teaspoon black pepper

⅛   teaspoon ground nutmeg

1. Preheat oven to 350°F. Lightly spray 9-inch glass pie plate with nonstick cooking spray.

2. Heat oil in medium skillet over medium-high heat. Add onion; cook 2 minutes or until soft, stirring occasionally. Add garlic; cook 1 minute. Stir in spinach and ham. Spread mixture evenly in prepared pie plate.

3. Combine milk, eggs, ¼ cup cheese, basil, pepper and nutmeg in medium bowl; whisk to blend. Pour mixture over spinach mixture. Bake 50 minutes or until knife inserted into center comes out clean. Sprinkle with remaining 2 tablespoons cheese. Cut evenly into six wedges.

nutritionals

Serving Size: *1 wedge*, Calories: *250*, Total Fat: *14g*, Saturated Fat: *6g*, Cholesterol: *170mg*, Sodium: *660mg*, Carbohydrate: *11g*, Dietary Fiber: *2g*, Sugar: *6g*, Protein: *18g*

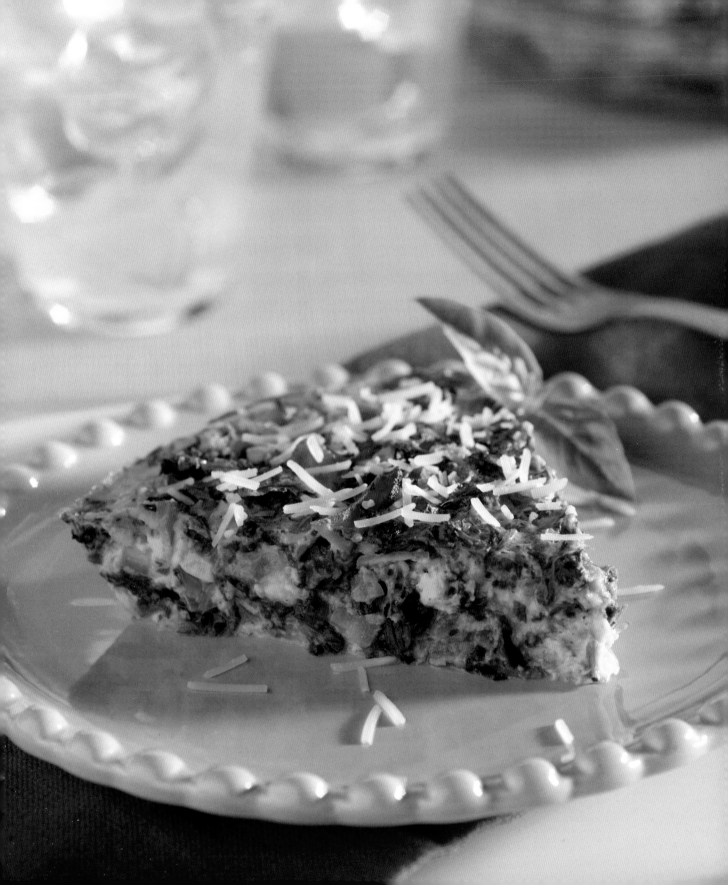

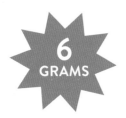

6 GRAMS

KIWI & STRAWBERRIES WITH PINE NUTS

makes 4 servings

2 kiwi fruits

1½ cups fresh strawberries

1 tablespoon fresh orange juice

1 tablespoon pine nuts,* toasted

*To toast pine nuts, cook and stir in small skillet over medium heat 3 minutes or until lightly browned.

1. Peel kiwis; slice each into 6 thin rounds. Arrange 3 slices kiwi on four dessert plates.

2. Wash, hull and slice strawberries. Arrange strawberries evenly over kiwi slices. Drizzle orange juice evenly over each plate. Top evenly with pine nuts.

nutritionals

Serving Size: *1 plate*, Calories: *90*, Total Fat: *5g*, Saturated Fat: *1g*, Cholesterol: *0mg*, Sodium: *0mg*, Carbohydrate: *11g*, Dietary Fiber: *3g*, Sugar: *6g*, Protein: *2g*

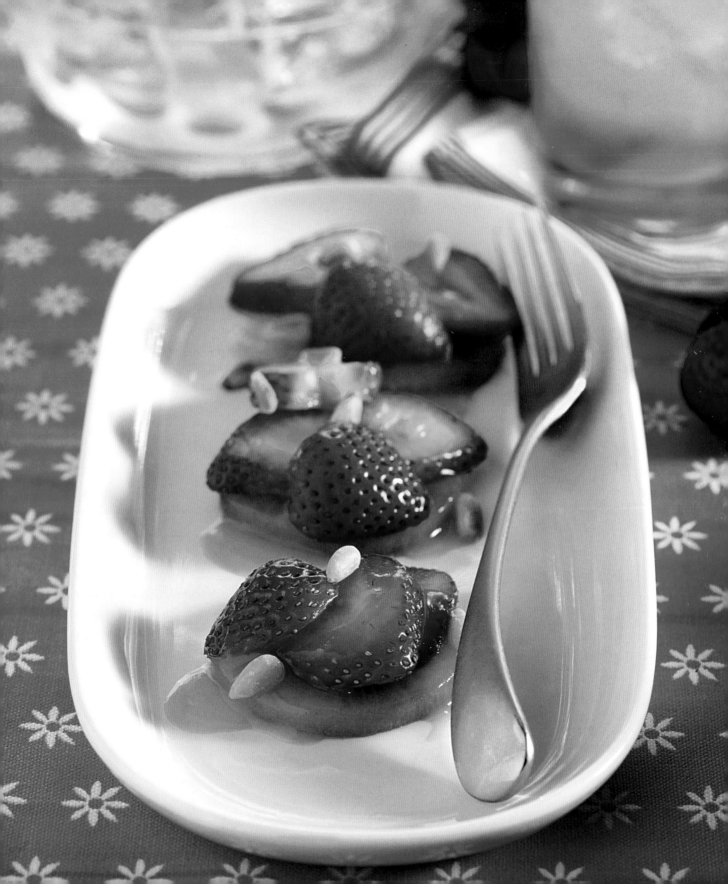

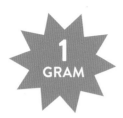

1 GRAM

SCRAMBLED EGG & ZUCCHINI PIE

makes 2 servings

2   eggs

2   tablespoons grated Parmesan or Cheddar cheese

¼   teaspoon salt

2   teaspoons butter

1   small zucchini, diced

1. Preheat oven to 350°F.

2. Whisk eggs in small bowl; stir in cheese and salt.

3. Melt butter in small nonstick ovenproof skillet over medium-high heat. Add zucchini; cook and stir 2 to 3 minutes or until crisp-tender.

4. Reduce heat to low; stir egg mixture into skillet with zucchini. Cook without stirring 4 to 5 minutes or until eggs begin to set around edge.

5. Transfer skillet to oven and bake 5 minutes or until eggs are set. Cut in half evenly to serve.

nutritionals

Serving Size: *½ pie*, Calories: *140*, Total Fat: *11g*, Saturated Fat: *5g*, Cholesterol: *235mg*, Sodium: *530mg*, Carbohydrate: *3g*, Dietary Fiber: *1g*, Sugar: *1g*, Protein: *11g*

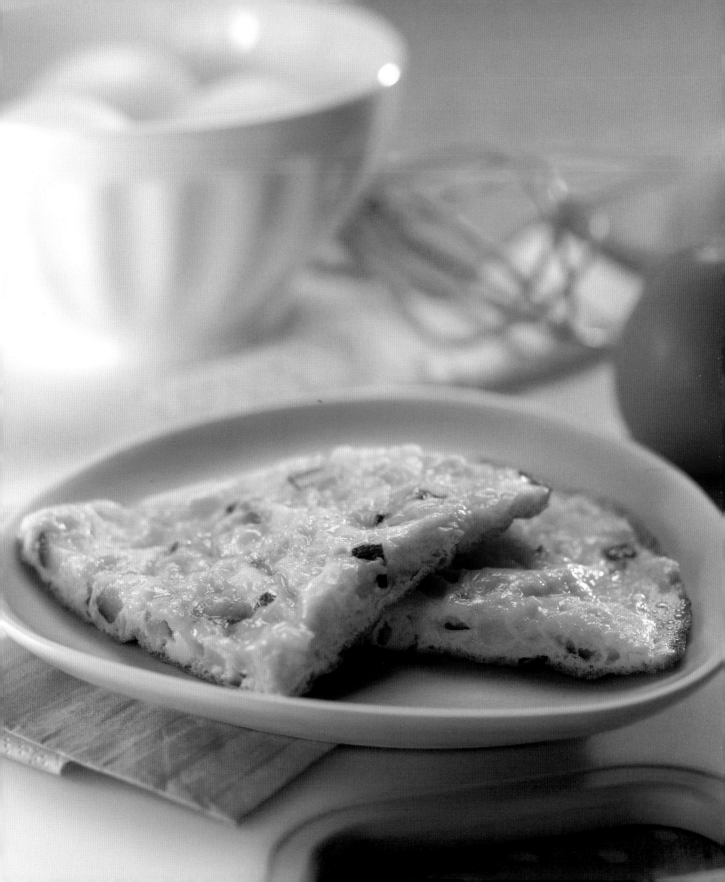

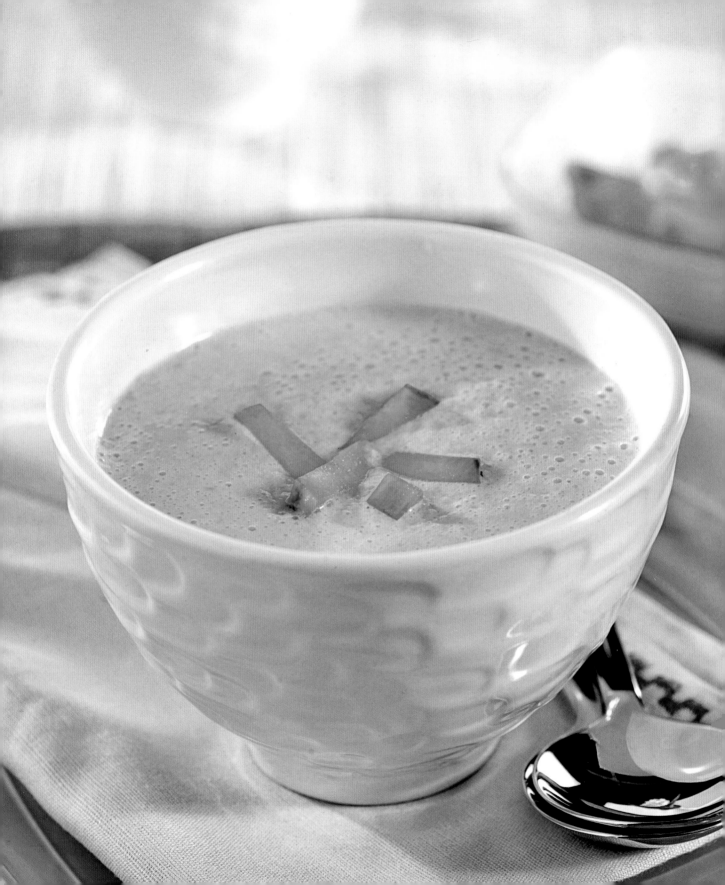

SOUPS

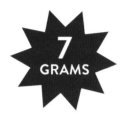

7 GRAMS

CHILLED CANTALOUPE SOUP

makes 4 servings

½ medium to large cantaloupe, rind removed, seeded and cut into cubes

¼ cup plain nonfat Greek yogurt

¾ cup half-and-half

Salt and white pepper

Slivered cantaloupe (optional)

1. Place cubed cantaloupe in food processor or blender; process until smooth. Add yogurt; process until blended.

2. Pour cantaloupe mixture into medium bowl; stir in half-and-half. Season with salt and pepper to taste. Refrigerate until ready to serve. Garnish with slivered cantaloupe.

SUMMER HONEYDEW SOUP: Substitute ½ medium honeydew melon for cantaloupe.

TIP: This refreshing soup makes a great first course, light lunch or breakfast.

---

nutritionals

Serving Size: *about ½ cup*, Calories: *90*, Total Fat: *5g*, Saturated Fat: *3g*, Cholesterol: *15mg*, Sodium: *35mg*, Carbohydrate: *8g*, Dietary Fiber: *1g*, Sugar: *7g*, Protein: *3g*

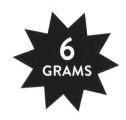

6 GRAMS

SHRIMP GAZPACHO

makes 2 servings

1 teaspoon olive oil

½ pound medium shrimp, peeled and deveined (with tails on)

⅛ teaspoon black pepper

⅛ teaspoon salt

3 plum tomatoes, chopped (about 1½ cups)

¼ small red onion, chopped

1 clove garlic, chopped

¼ cucumber, peeled and chopped

¼ cup finely chopped jarred roasted red peppers, divided

¾ cup tomato juice

1 tablespoon red wine vinegar

1. Heat oil in medium nonstick skillet over high heat. Season shrimp with black pepper and salt. Add to skillet; cook 3 minutes or until browned on both sides and opaque in center. Transfer to plate.

2. Combine tomatoes, onion, garlic, cucumber and half of roasted peppers in food processor; process until blended. Add tomato juice and vinegar; process until smooth.

3. Divide tomato mixture among bowls; top with shrimp and remaining roasted peppers.

---

nutritionals

Serving Size: *1½ cups*, Calories: *150*, Total Fat: *4g*, Saturated Fat: *1g*, Cholesterol: *145mg*, Sodium: *1150mg*, Carbohydrate: *12g*, Dietary Fiber: *2g*, Sugar: *6g*, Protein: *18g*

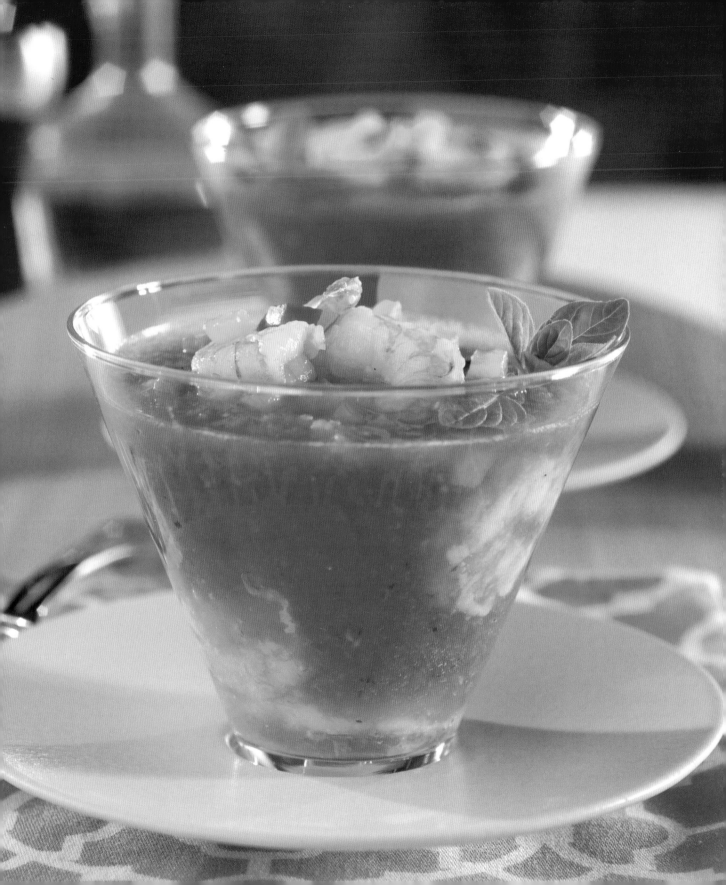

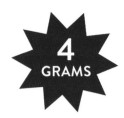

4 GRAMS

CHILLED FRESH TOMATO BASIL SOUP

makes 4 servings

3   medium tomatoes, diced

1   cup finely chopped green
     bell pepper

½   medium cucumber, peeled,
     seeded and finely chopped

¼   cup chopped fresh basil

¼   cup finely chopped
     peperoncinis

1   cup water

3   tablespoons red wine
     vinegar

½   teaspoon salt

2   tablespoons chopped fresh
     parsley

2   tablespoons extra virgin
     olive oil

Combine tomatoes, bell pepper, cucumber, basil, peperoncinis, water, vinegar, salt, parsley and oil in medium bowl; stir to blend. Cover; refrigerate 30 minutes.

---

nutritionals

Serving Size: *about 1 cup*, Calories: *100*, Total Fat: *7g*, Saturated Fat: *1g*, Cholesterol: *0mg*, Sodium: *490mg*, Carbohydrate: *7g*, Dietary Fiber: *2g*, Sugar: *4g*, Protein: *2g*

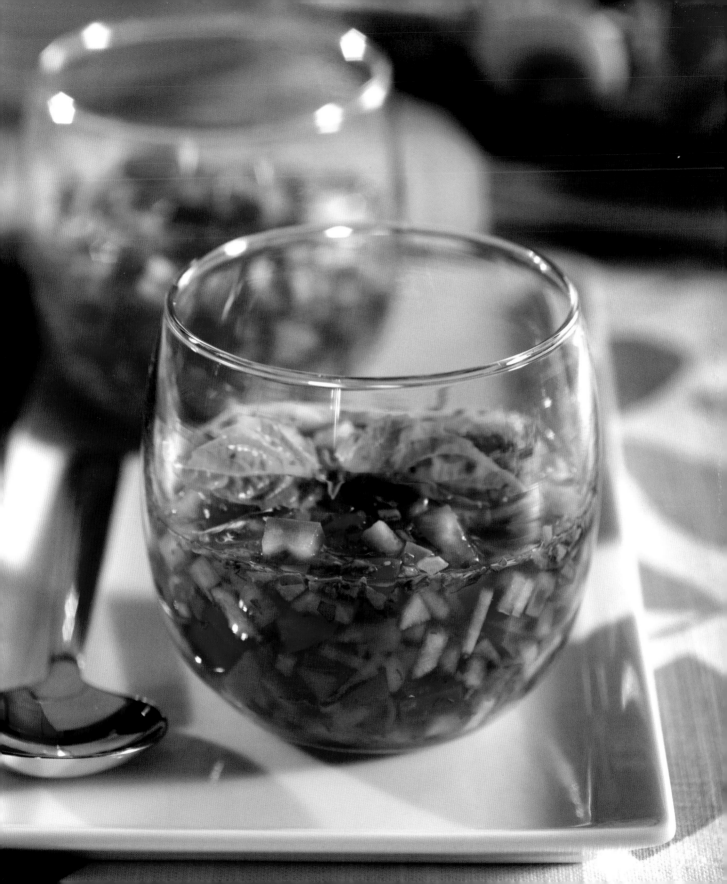

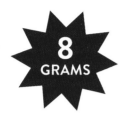

8 GRAMS

MINTED MELON SOUP

makes 4 servings

1 cup water

1½ cups fresh mint, including stems

2 fresh basil leaves

1½ cups diced cantaloupe

4 teaspoons lemon juice, divided

1½ cups diced seeded watermelon

Sprigs fresh mint (optional)

1. Bring water to a boil in small saucepan over medium heat. Add 1½ cups mint and basil; simmer 10 minutes or until reduced by two-thirds. Remove from heat; cover and let stand at least 2 hours or until cool. Strain mint syrup; set aside.

2. Place cantaloupe in food processor or blender; process until smooth. Add 2 tablespoons mint syrup and 2 teaspoons lemon juice; process until well mixed. Pour into airtight container. Cover and refrigerate until cold. Repeat procedure with watermelon, 2 teaspoons mint syrup and remaining 2 teaspoons lemon juice. Discard any remaining mint syrup.

3. To serve, simultaneously pour ¼ cup of each melon soup, side by side, into serving bowl. Garnish with mint sprigs. Repeat with remaining soup.

---

nutritionals

Serving Size: ½ cup, Calories: 45, Total Fat: 0g, Saturated Fat: 0g, Cholesterol: 0mg, Sodium: 15mg, Carbohydrate: 11g, Dietary Fiber: 2g, Sugar: 8g, Protein: 1g

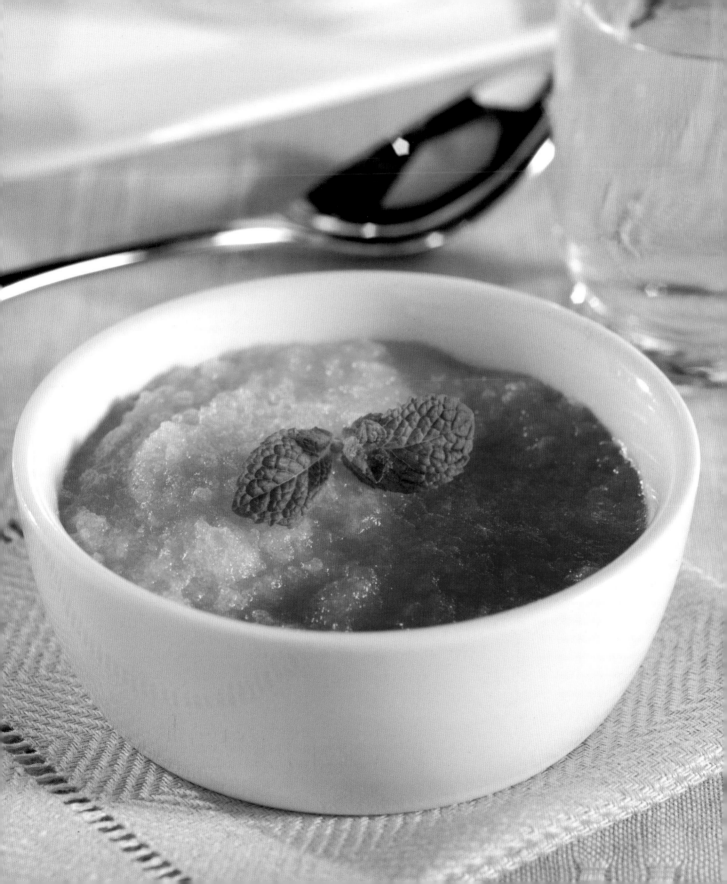

CHICKEN BROTH

makes about 10 cups

1   cut-up whole chicken (about 5 pounds)

2   medium onions, cut into wedges

2   medium carrots, halved

2   stalks celery, including leaves, cut into halves

1   clove garlic, crushed

1   bay leaf

6   sprigs fresh parsley

8   black peppercorns

½   teaspoon dried thyme

3   quarts cold water

1. Place chicken, onions, carrots, celery, garlic, bay leaf, parsley, peppercorns, thyme and water into stockpot or 6-quart Dutch oven. Bring to a boil over high heat. Reduce heat to medium-low. Simmer, uncovered, 3 to 4 hours, skimming foam that rises to surface.

2. Remove broth from heat; cool slightly. Remove large bones. Strain broth through large sieve or colander lined with several layers of damp cheesecloth; discard bones and vegetables.

3. Use immediately or refrigerate in tightly covered container up to 2 days. Or freeze broth in batches in freezer containers for several months.

HINT: Roasting poultry in a 450°F oven before simmering produces a broth that is richer in flavor and color.

NOTE: Broth is economical to make, because bones and tough cuts of meat can be used.

VEGETABLE BROTH

makes about 7 cups

2 medium onions

2 tablespoons vegetable oil

2 leeks, cleaned and coarsely chopped

3 stalks celery, cut into 2-inch pieces

8 cups cold water

6 medium carrots, cut into 1-inch pieces

1 turnip, peeled and cut into chunks (optional)

2 cloves garlic, crushed

4 sprigs fresh parsley

1 teaspoon dried thyme

2 bay leaves

¼ teaspoon black pepper

1. Trim tops and roots from onions, leaving most of dried outer skin intact; cut into wedges.

2. Heat oil in stockpot or Dutch oven over medium-high heat. Add onions, leeks and celery; cook and stir 5 minutes or until vegetables are limp but not browned. Add water, carrots, turnip, if desired, garlic, parsley, thyme, bay leaves and pepper; bring to a boil over high heat. Reduce heat to medium-low. Simmer, uncovered, 1½ hours.

3. Remove from heat; cool slightly. Strain stock through large sieve or colander, pressing vegetables lightly with slotted spoon to remove excess liquid. Discard vegetables.

4. Use immediately or refrigerate in tightly covered container up to 2 days. Or freeze broth in batches in freezer containers for several months.

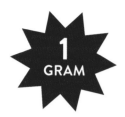
1 GRAM

SHRIMP, MUSHROOM AND OMELET SOUP

makes 6 servings

10 to 12 dried shiitake mushrooms (about 1 ounce)

3 eggs

1 tablespoon chopped fresh chives or minced green onion tops

2 teaspoons vegetable oil

3 cans (about 14 ounces each) chicken broth

2 tablespoons oyster sauce

12 ounces medium raw shrimp, peeled and deveined

3 cups lightly packed fresh spinach leaves, washed and stemmed

1 tablespoon lime juice

Red pepper flakes and lime peel (optional)

1. Place mushrooms in small bowl; cover with hot water. Let stand 30 minutes or until caps are soft.

2. Meanwhile, beat eggs and chives in small bowl until blended. Heat oil in large skillet over medium heat. Pour egg mixture into pan. Reduce heat to medium. Cover; cook 2 minutes or until set on bottom. Slide spatula under omelet. Lift omelet and tilt pan to allow uncooked egg to flow under. Cook 2 minutes. When cool enough to handle, roll up omelet; cut into ¼-inch-wide strips.

3. Drain mushrooms; squeeze out excess water. Remove and discard stems. Slice caps into thin strips.

4. Combine mushrooms, broth and oyster sauce in large saucepan. Cover; bring to a boil over high heat. Reduce heat to medium. Cook 5 minutes. Add shrimp; cook 2 minutes or until shrimp turn pink and opaque. Add omelet strips and spinach; remove from heat. Cover; let stand 1 to 2 minutes or until spinach wilts slightly. Stir in lime juice. Ladle soup into bowls. Sprinkle with red pepper flakes and lime peel, if desired.

---

nutritionals

Serving Size: *about 1¼ cups*, Calories: *120*, Total Fat: *5g*, Saturated Fat: *1g*, Cholesterol: *165mg*, Sodium: *1350mg*, Carbohydrate: *7g*, Dietary Fiber: *1g*, Sugar: *1g*, Protein: *12g*

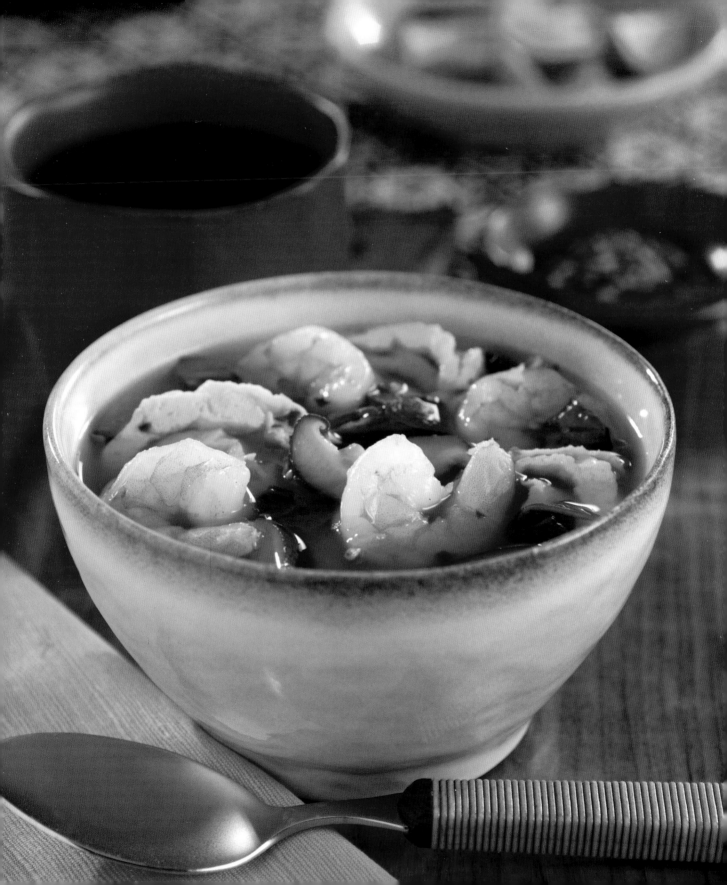

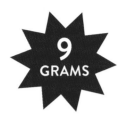

9 GRAMS

CARROT & CORIANDER SOUP

makes 4 servings

¼ cup (½ stick) butter

4 cups grated carrots (about 1 pound)

1 cup finely chopped onion

3 cups chicken broth

2 tablespoons lemon juice

1½ teaspoons ground coriander

1½ teaspoons ground cumin

1 clove garlic, minced

2 tablespoons finely chopped fresh coriander (cilantro)

Salt and black pepper

1. Melt butter in medium saucepan over medium-high heat. Add carrots and onion; cook and stir 5 minutes or until softened. Add broth, lemon juice, ground coriander, cumin and garlic. Bring to a boil over high heat. Reduce heat to low. Cover; simmer 25 to 30 minutes.

2. Process soup in batches in food processor or blender until smooth. Stir in fresh coriander. Season with salt and pepper.

nutritionals

Serving Size: *about 1½ cups*, Calories: *190*, Total Fat: *12g*, Saturated Fat: *7g*, Cholesterol: *30mg*, Sodium: *560mg*, Carbohydrate: *19g*, Dietary Fiber: *4g*, Sugar: *9g*, Protein: *3g*

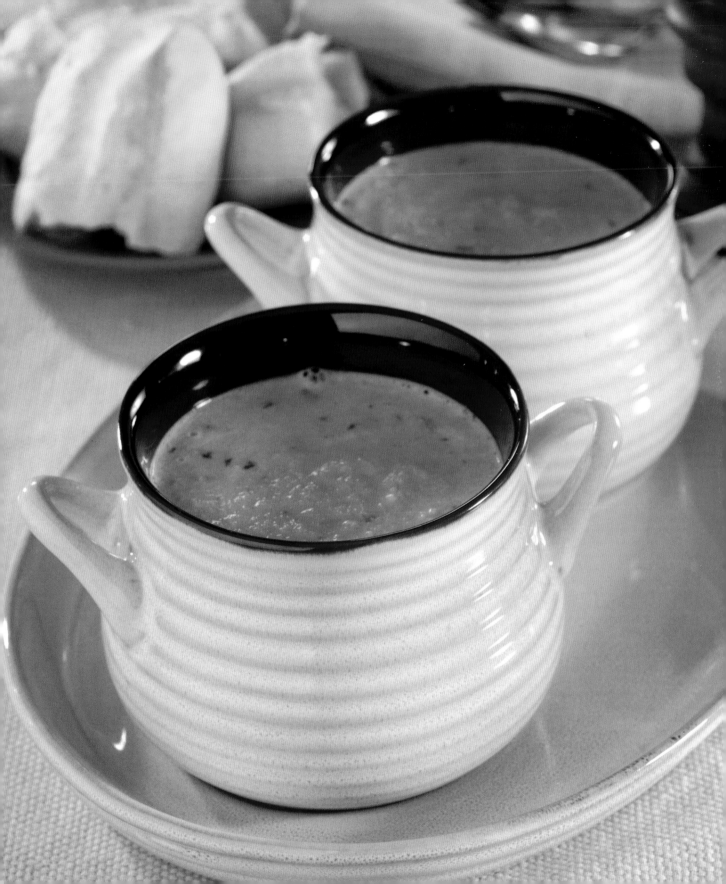

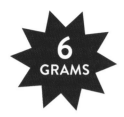

6 GRAMS

GARLIC LENTIL SOUP WITH MUSHROOMS AND GREENS

makes 10 servings

¾ cup olive oil

1 whole head garlic

2 tablespoons fresh rosemary

3 medium stalks celery, diced

2 medium onions, chopped

1 bag (16 ounces) green lentils

12 fresh sage leaves

12 cups vegetable broth

1 package (8 ounces) mushrooms

8 ounces kale, spinach or Swiss chard, coarsely chopped

6 tablespoons grated Parmesan or Romano cheese (optional)

Chopped fresh Italian parsley (optional)

SLOW COOKER DIRECTIONS

1. Place oil, garlic and rosemary in small bowl; cover with foil. Place bowl in slow cooker. Cover; cook on HIGH 1½ hours. Drain, reserving garlic oil and garlic cloves separately; refrigerate. Discard rosemary. (This portion of the recipe can be prepared up to 2 days in advance.)

2. Heat 2 tablespoons garlic oil in large skillet over medium-high heat. Add celery and onions; cook and stir until onions caramelize. Remove to slow cooker. Add lentils, sage, broth and mushrooms. Cover; cook on LOW 8 hours or on HIGH 4 hours.

3. Heat 3 to 4 tablespoons garlic oil in skillet over medium heat. Add kale; cook and stir just until tender. Stir kale into soup. Sprinkle with cheese and parsley, if desired.

nutritionals

Serving Size: *2½ cups*, Calories: *280*, Total Fat: *5g*, Saturated Fat: *1g*, Cholesterol: *0mg*, Sodium: *1020mg*, Carbohydrate: *44g*, Dietary Fiber: *11g*, Sugar: *6g*, Protein: *16g*

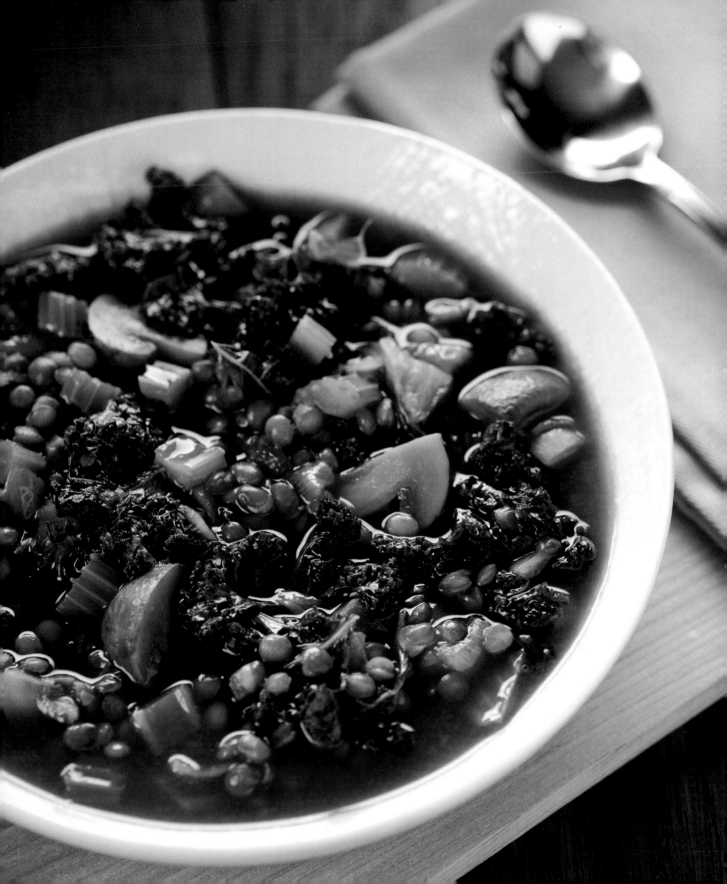

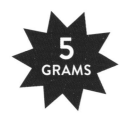

5 GRAMS

TOMATO-HERB SOUP

makes 4 servings

1   can (about 14 ounces) diced tomatoes

1   can (about 14 ounces) chicken broth

1   cup sliced bell peppers

1   cup frozen green beans

½   cup water

1   to 2 teaspoons dried oregano

1   teaspoon dried basil

⅛   teaspoon red pepper flakes (optional)

Combine tomatoes, broth, bell peppers, green beans, water, oregano, basil and red pepper flakes, if desired, in large saucepan. Bring to a boil over medium-high heat. Reduce heat to medium-low. Simmer, covered, 20 minutes or until beans are tender.

---

nutritionals

Serving Size: *about 1 cup*, Calories: *50*, Total Fat: *0g*, Saturated Fat: *0g*, Cholesterol: *0mg*, Sodium: *640mg*, Carbohydrate: *10g*, Dietary Fiber: *3g*, Sugar: *5g*, Protein: *2g*

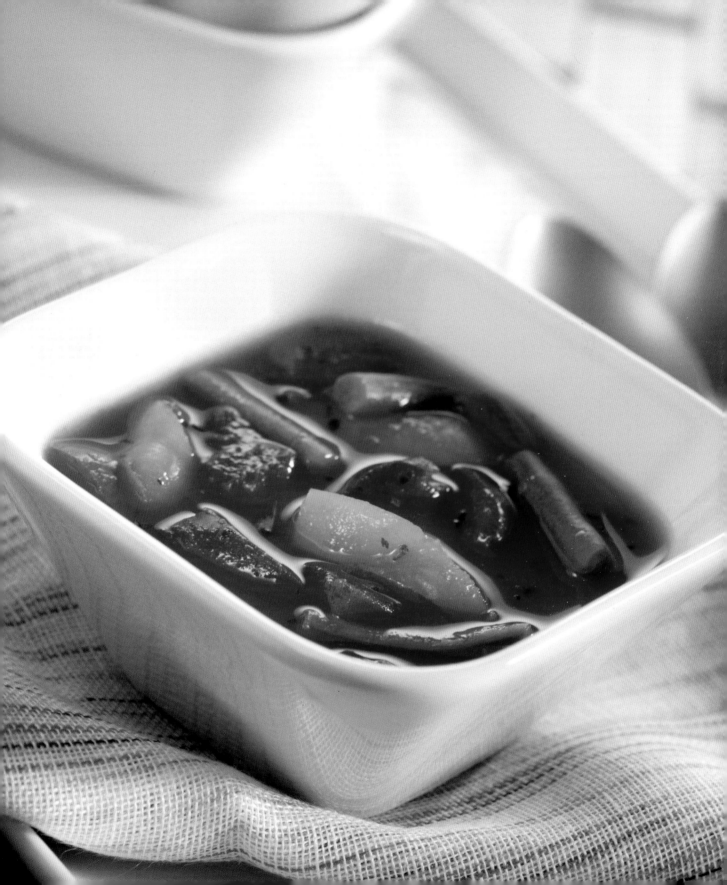

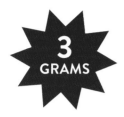

3 GRAMS

CHICKEN BARLEY SOUP

makes 6 servings

1   teaspoon olive oil

¾   cup chopped onion

¾   cup chopped carrot

¾   cup chopped celery

1   package (8 ounces) sliced
      mushrooms

2   cloves garlic, minced

4   cups chicken broth

1   cup chopped cooked
      chicken

½   cup uncooked quick-
      cooking barley

¼   teaspoon dried thyme

¼   teaspoon black pepper

1   bay leaf

     Juice of 1 lemon

     Chopped fresh parsley
      (optional)

1. Heat oil in Dutch oven over medium-high heat.
   Add onion, carrot, celery, mushrooms and garlic;
   cook 5 minutes.

2. Add broth, chicken, barley, thyme, pepper and bay
   leaf; bring to a boil. Reduce heat to medium. Cover;
   simmer 25 minutes or until vegetables are tender.

3. Remove and discard bay leaf. Stir in lemon juice and
   sprinkle with parsley, if desired.

nutritionals

Serving Size: *about 1¼ cups*, Calories: *140*, Total Fat:
2g, Saturated Fat: *0g*, Cholesterol: *20mg*, Sodium:
690mg, Carbohydrate: *19g*, Dietary Fiber: *4g*,
Sugar: *3g*, Protein: *11g*

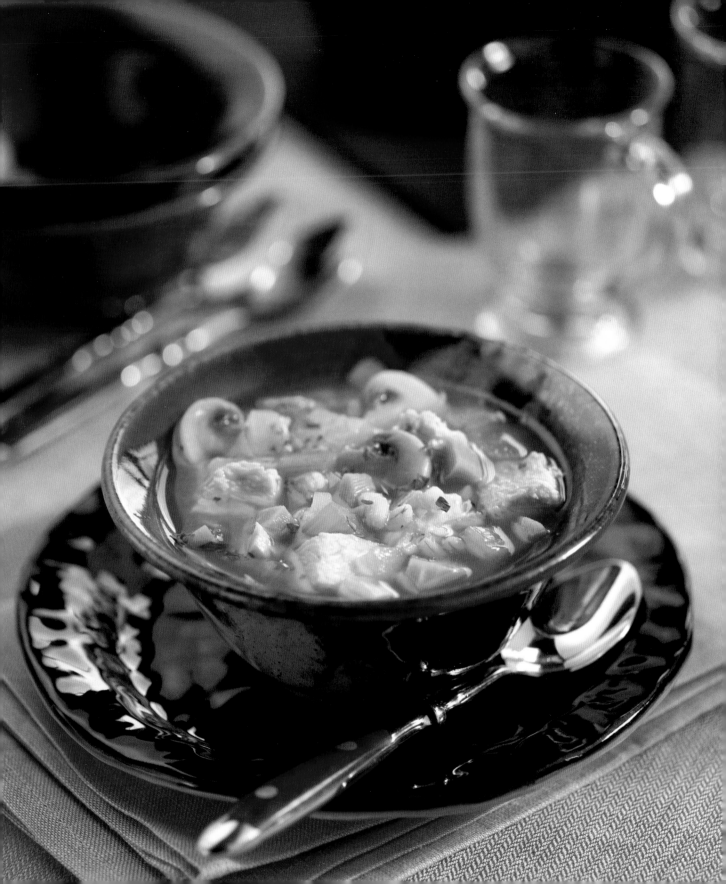

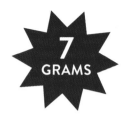

7 GRAMS

GROUNDNUT SOUP WITH GINGER AND CILANTRO

makes 6 servings

1 tablespoon vegetable oil

1½ cups chopped onion

1 medium clove garlic, minced

2 teaspoons chili powder

1 teaspoon ground cumin

¼ teaspoon red pepper flakes

3 cups chicken broth

1 can (about 14 ounces) diced tomatoes, undrained

8 ounces sweet potatoes, peeled and cut into ½-inch cubes

1 medium carrot, cut into ½-inch pieces

1 cup salted peanuts

1 tablespoon grated fresh ginger

¼ cup chopped fresh cilantro

1. Heat oil in large saucepan over medium-high heat. Add onion; cook and stir 4 minutes or until translucent. Add garlic, chili powder, cumin and red pepper flakes; cook and stir 15 seconds.

2. Add broth, tomatoes, sweet potatoes and carrot; bring to a boil over high heat. Reduce heat to medium. Cover tightly; simmer 25 minutes or until vegetables are tender, stirring occasionally. Remove from heat. Stir in peanuts and ginger. Cool slightly.

3. Working in batches, process soup in blender or food processor until smooth. Return to saucepan. Heat over medium-high heat 2 minutes or until heated through. Sprinkle cilantro over each serving.

---

nutritionals

Serving Size: *about 1¼ cups*, Calories: *230*, Total Fat: *15g*, Saturated Fat: *2g*, Cholesterol: *0mg*, Sodium: *800mg*, Carbohydrate: *20g*, Dietary Fiber: *4g*, Sugar: *7g*, Protein: *9g*

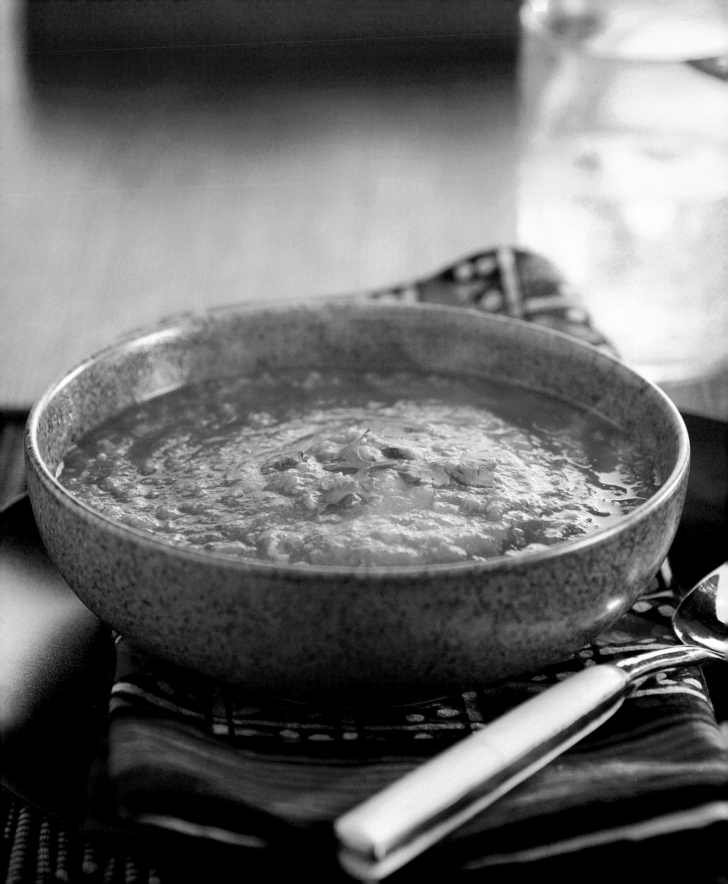

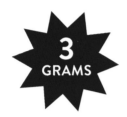

3 GRAMS

BUTTERNUT SQUASH AND MILLET SOUP

makes 6 servings

1   red bell pepper

1   teaspoon canola oil

2¼ cups diced butternut squash *or* 1 package (10 ounces) frozen diced butternut squash

1   medium red onion, chopped

1   teaspoon curry powder

½   teaspoon smoked paprika

½   teaspoon salt

⅛   teaspoon black pepper

2   cups chicken broth

2   boneless skinless chicken breasts (about 4 ounces each), cooked and chopped

1   cup cooked millet

1. Place bell pepper on rack in broiler pan 3 to 5 inches from heat source or hold over open gas flame on long-handled metal fork. Turn bell pepper often until blistered and charred on all sides. Transfer to medium resealable food storage bag; seal bag and let stand 15 to 20 minutes to loosen skin. Remove loosened skin with paring knife. Cut off top and scrape out seeds; discard. Chop remaining bell pepper into pieces.

2. Heat oil in large saucepan over high heat. Add squash, bell pepper pieces and onion; cook and stir 5 minutes. Add curry powder, paprika, salt and black pepper. Pour in broth; bring to a boil. Cover; cook 7 to 10 minutes or until vegetables are tender.

3. Purée soup in saucepan with hand-held immersion blender or in batches in food processor or blender. Return soup to saucepan. Stir in chicken and millet; cook until heated through.

---

nutritionals

Serving Size: *1⅓ cups*, Calories: *140*, Total Fat: *3g*, Saturated Fat: *1g*, Cholesterol: *30mg*, Sodium: *550mg*, Carbohydrate: *17g*, Dietary Fiber: *2g*, Sugar: *3g*, Protein: *14g*

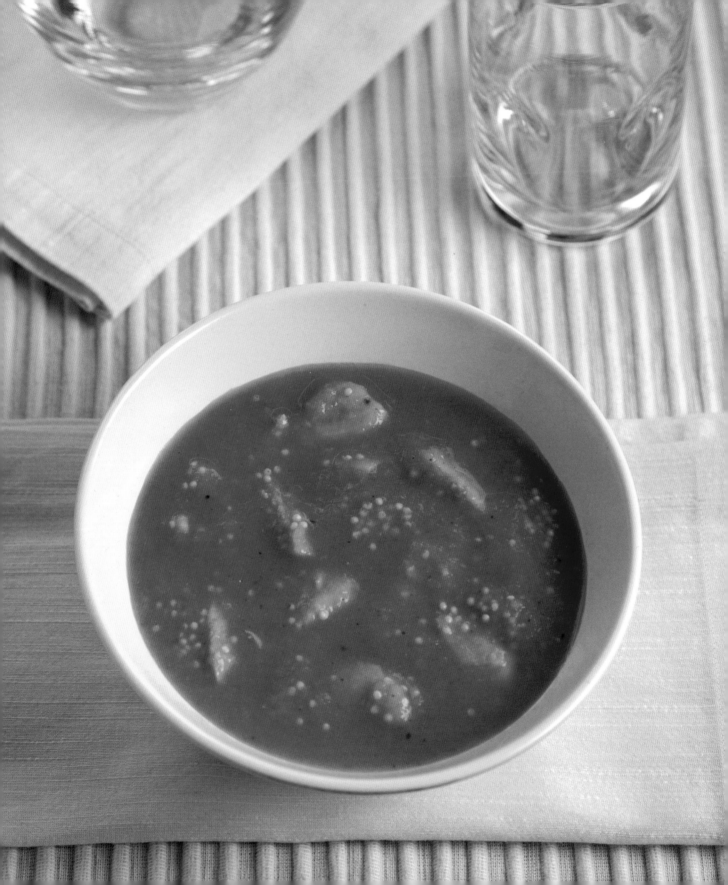

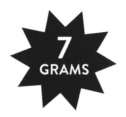

7 GRAMS

VEGETABLE SOUP WITH BEANS

makes 6 servings

4   cups vegetable broth

1   can (about 15 ounces) cannellini beans, rinsed and drained

1   can (about 14 ounces) diced tomatoes

16 baby carrots

1   medium onion, chopped

1   ounce dried oyster mushrooms, chopped

3   tablespoons tomato paste

2   teaspoons garlic powder

1   teaspoon dried basil

1   teaspoon dried oregano

½   teaspoon dried rosemary

½   teaspoon dried marjoram

½   teaspoon dried sage

½   teaspoon dried thyme

¼   teaspoon black pepper

SLOW COOKER DIRECTIONS

Combine broth, beans, tomatoes, carrots, onion, mushrooms, tomato paste, garlic powder, basil, oregano, rosemary, marjoram, sage, thyme and pepper in slow cooker; stir to blend. Cover; cook on LOW 8 hours or on HIGH 4 to 5 hours.

nutritionals

Serving Size: *about 1½ cups*, Calories: *130*, Total Fat: *0g*, Saturated Fat: *0g*, Cholesterol: *0mg*, Sodium: *320mg*, Carbohydrate: *24g*, Dietary Fiber: *6g*, Sugar: *7g*, Protein: *7g*

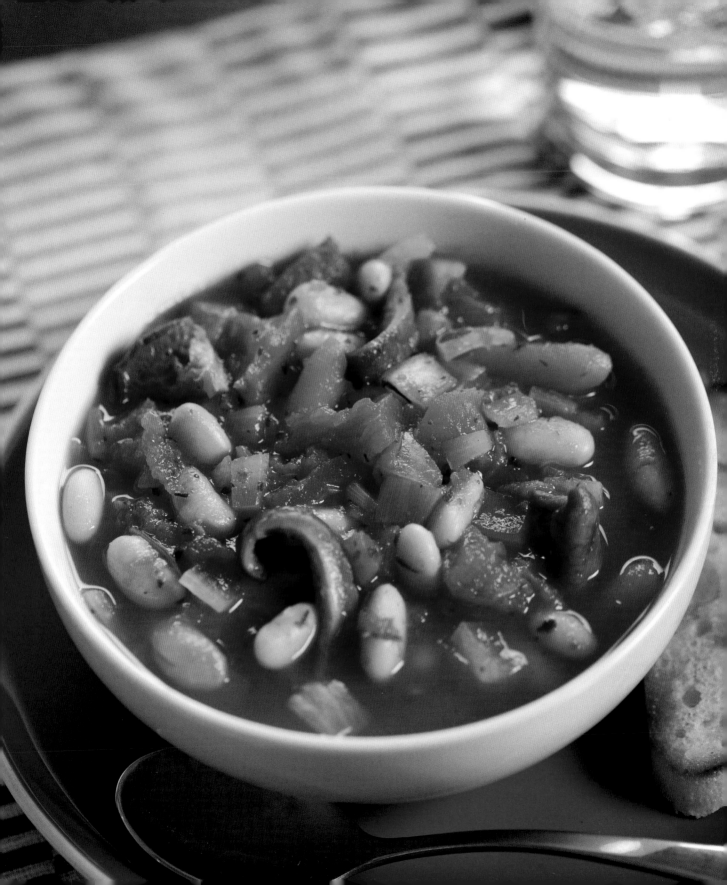

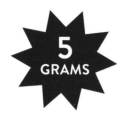

5 GRAMS

SKILLET CHICKEN SOUP

makes 6 servings

1 teaspoon paprika

½ teaspoon salt

¼ teaspoon black pepper

¾ pound boneless skinless chicken breasts or thighs, cut into ¾-inch pieces

2 teaspoons vegetable oil

1 large onion, chopped

1 red bell pepper, cut into ½-inch pieces

3 cloves garlic, minced

3 cups chicken broth

1 can (19 ounces) cannellini beans or small white beans, rinsed and drained

3 cups sliced savoy or napa cabbage

1. Combine paprika, salt and black pepper in medium bowl; stir to blend. Add chicken; toss to coat.

2. Heat oil in large deep nonstick skillet over medium-high heat. Add chicken, onion, bell pepper and garlic; cook and stir 8 minutes or until chicken is cooked through.

3. Add broth and beans; bring to a simmer. Cover and simmer 5 minutes. Stir in cabbage; cover and simmer 3 minutes or until cabbage is wilted. Ladle evenly into six shallow bowls.

TIP: Savoy cabbage, also called curly cabbage, is round with pale green crinkled leaves. Napa cabbage is also known as Chinese cabbage and is elongated with light green stalks.

nutritionals

Serving Size: *about 1½ cups*, Calories: *190*, Total Fat: *3g*, Saturated Fat: *1g*, Cholesterol: *40mg*, Sodium: *950mg*, Carbohydrate: *21g*, Dietary Fiber: *6g*, Sugar: *5g*, Protein: *20g*

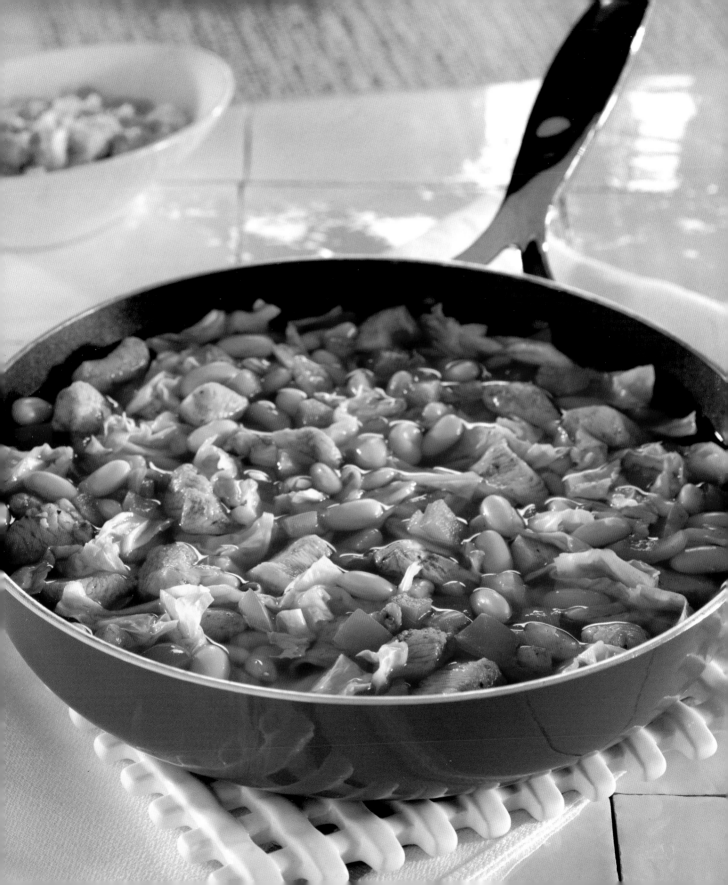

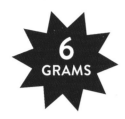

6 GRAMS

ITALIAN FISH SOUP

makes 4 servings

1 can (about 14 ounces) Italian seasoned diced tomatoes

1 can (about 14 ounces) chicken broth

1 small fennel bulb, chopped (about 1 cup), reserve fennel fronds for garnish

3 cloves garlic, minced

1 tablespoon olive oil

½ teaspoon saffron threads, crushed (optional)

½ teaspoon dried basil

¼ teaspoon red pepper flakes

½ pound (8 ounces) skinless halibut or cod fillets, cut into 1-inch chunks

½ pound (8 ounces) raw medium shrimp, peeled and deveined

SLOW COOKER DIRECTIONS

1. Combine tomatoes, broth, chopped fennel bulb, garlic, oil, saffron, if desired, basil and red pepper flakes in slow cooker. Cover; cook on LOW 4 to 5 hours or on HIGH 2½ to 3 hours or until fennel is tender.

2. Stir in halibut and shrimp. Cover; cook on HIGH 15 to 30 minutes or until shrimp are pink and opaque and fish begins to flake when tested with a fork. Ladle soup into shallow bowls. Garnish with reserved fennel fronds.

nutritionals

Serving Size: *about 1½ cups*, Calories: *170*, Total Fat: *5g*, Saturated Fat: *1g*, Cholesterol: *100mg*, Sodium: *1060mg*, Carbohydrate: *11g*, Dietary Fiber: *3g*, Sugar: *6g*, Protein: *20g*

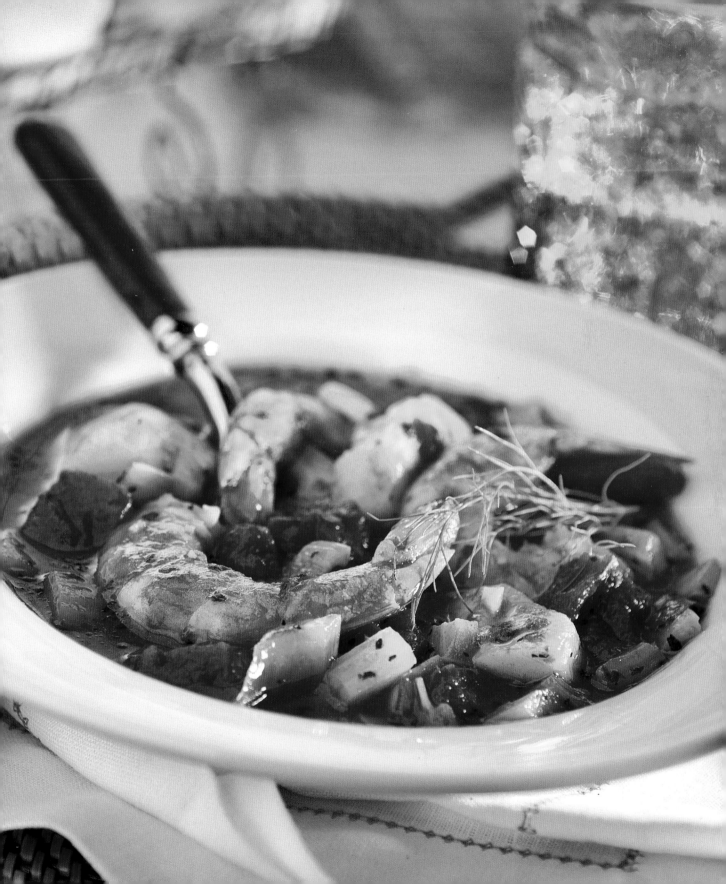

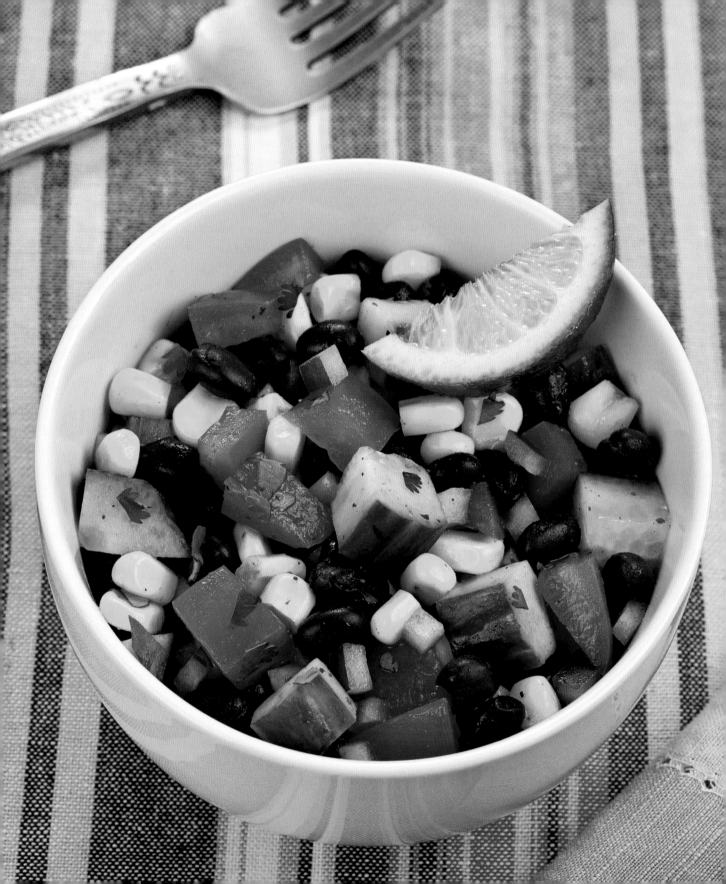

SALADS

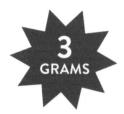

3 GRAMS

SOUTHWEST GAZPACHO SALAD

makes 4 servings

1 cup canned black beans, rinsed and drained

1 cup diced tomato

⅔ cup corn

½ cup diced cucumber

2 tablespoons diced red onion

1 tablespoon finely chopped fresh cilantro

3 tablespoons tomato juice

1 tablespoon lime juice

2 teaspoons extra virgin olive oil

½ teaspoon chili powder

¼ teaspoon salt

Pinch black pepper

1. Combine beans, tomato, corn, cucumber, onion and cilantro in large bowl; toss to blend.

2. Whisk tomato juice, lime juice, oil, chili powder, salt and pepper in small bowl. Pour over salad; toss to blend.

---

nutritionals

Serving Size: *about ¾ cup*, Calories: *110*, Total Fat: *3g*, Saturated Fat: *0g*, Cholesterol: *0mg*, Sodium: *530mg*, Carbohydrate: *18g*, Dietary Fiber: *4g*, Sugar: *3g*, Protein: *4g*

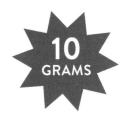

10 GRAMS

SPINACH SALAD WITH ORANGE-CHILI GLAZED SHRIMP

makes 6 servings

¾ cup orange juice, divided

5 cloves garlic, minced and divided

1 teaspoon chili powder

8 ounces large raw shrimp, peeled and deveined (with tails on)

1 tablespoon cider vinegar

2 teaspoons toasted sesame seeds*

1 teaspoon grated orange peel

1 teaspoon olive oil

⅛ teaspoon red pepper flakes

12 cups packed fresh spinach

1 large ripe mango or medium ripe papaya, peeled, cored and chopped

½ cup (2 ounces) crumbled feta cheese

*To toast sesame seeds, spread in small skillet. Shake skillet over medium-low heat 2 minutes or until seeds begin to pop and turn golden brown.

1. Combine ½ cup orange juice, 4 cloves garlic and chili powder in large nonstick skillet. Bring to a boil over high heat. Boil 3 minutes or until mixture just coats bottom of skillet.

2. Reduce heat to medium. Add shrimp; cook and stir 2 minutes or until shrimp are pink and opaque. (Add additional orange juice or water to keep shrimp moist, if necessary.) Set aside.

3. Combine remaining ¼ cup orange juice, vinegar, sesame seeds, remaining 1 clove garlic, orange peel, oil and red pepper flakes in small bowl; stir to blend. Set aside.

4. Place spinach leaves in large bowl; toss with dressing. Top with mango, cheese and shrimp.

---

nutritionals

Serving Size: *about 1 cup*, Calories: *140*, Total Fat: *4g*, Saturated Fat: *2g*, Cholesterol: *55mg*, Sodium: *400mg*, Carbohydrate: *16g*, Dietary Fiber: *4g*, Sugar: *10g*, Protein: *10g*

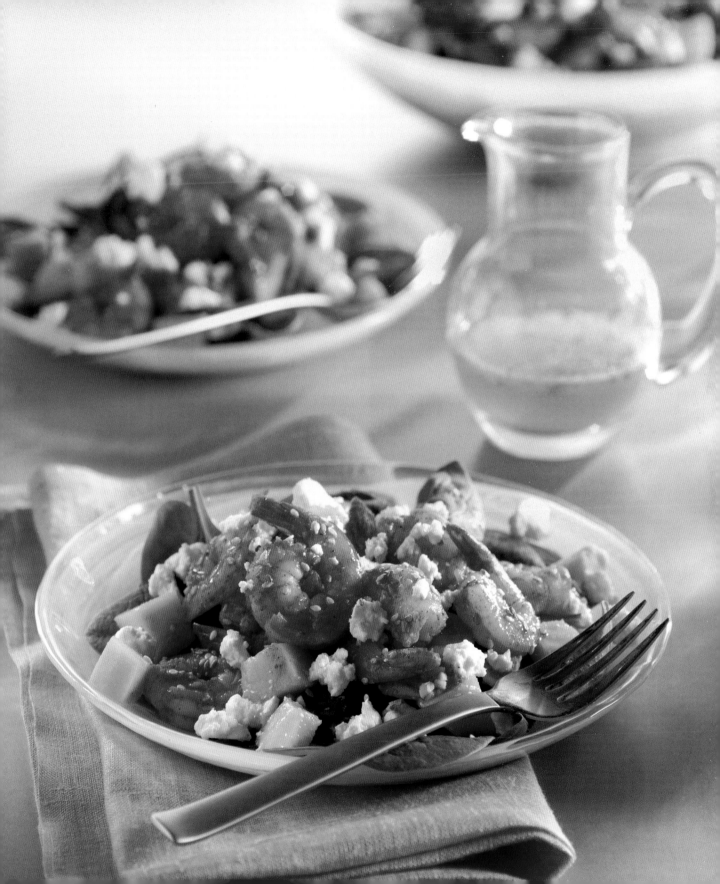

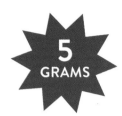

TUNA SALAD STUFFED PEPPERS >

makes 4 servings

2 cans (5 ounces each) albacore tuna packed in water, drained and flaked

2 large stalks celery, sliced diagonally

½ cup halved green grapes

½ cup (2 ounces) shredded sharp Cheddar cheese

⅓ cup mayonnaise

Salt and black pepper

2 red bell peppers, halved and seeded

Combine tuna, celery, grapes, cheese and mayonnaise in medium bowl; mix well. Season with salt and black pepper. Divide tuna mixture evenly among bell pepper halves.

_____

nutritionals

Serving Size: *1 bell pepper half*, Calories: *300*, Total Fat: *20g*, Saturated Fat: *6g*, Cholesterol: *45mg*, Sodium: *480mg*, Carbohydrate: *7g*, Dietary Fiber: *2g*, Sugar: *5g*, Protein: *20g*

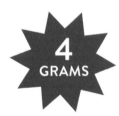

SPICED RICE AND CARROT SALAD

makes 2 servings

⅔ cup cooked brown rice, chilled

2 medium carrots, shredded

1 green onion, chopped

1 teaspoon white wine vinegar

1 teaspoon canola oil

1 teaspoon Chinese chili-garlic sauce

Salt and black pepper

Combine rice, carrots and green onion in medium bowl. Whisk vinegar, oil, chili-garlic sauce, salt and pepper in small bowl until well blended. Stir into rice mixture.

_____

nutritionals

Serving Size: *½ of recipe*, Calories: *120*, Total Fat: *3g*, Saturated Fat: *0g*, Cholesterol: *0mg*, Sodium: *90mg*, Carbohydrate: *22g*, Dietary Fiber: *3g*, Sugar: *4g*, Protein: *2g*

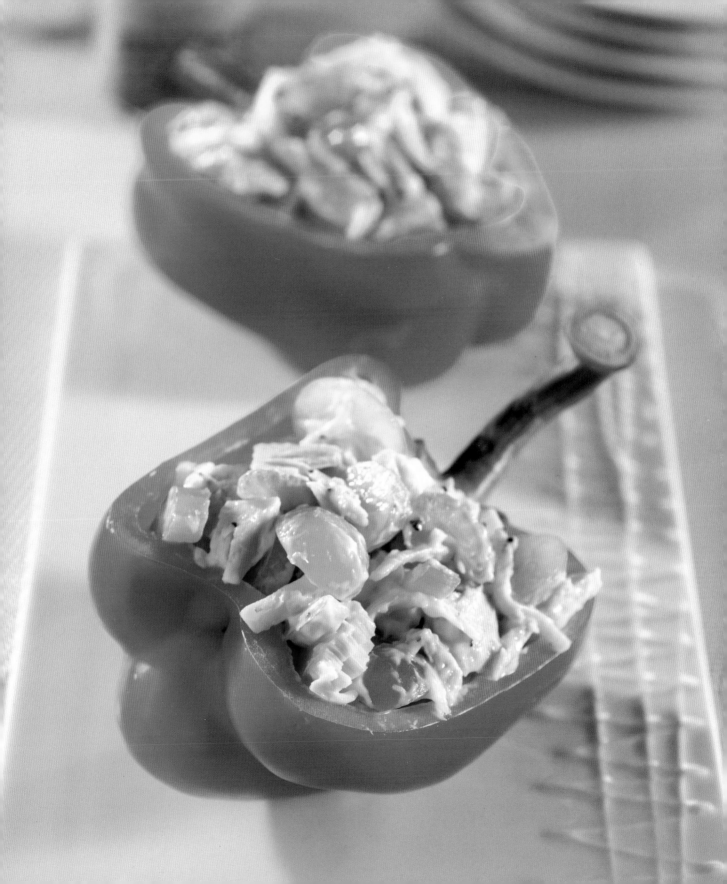

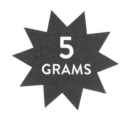
5 GRAMS

SUMMER SZECHUAN TOFU SALAD

makes 4 servings

¼ cup soy sauce

1 tablespoon canola or peanut oil

1 tablespoon dark sesame oil

1 teaspoon minced fresh ginger

½ teaspoon hot pepper sauce or more to taste

1 package (14 ounces) extra-firm tofu

4 cups baby spinach leaves

4 cups sliced napa cabbage or romaine lettuce leaves

2 cups diagonally halved fresh sugar snap peas or snow peas

1 cup matchstick-size carrots

1 cup fresh bean sprouts

¼ cup dry-roasted peanuts or toasted slivered almonds

Chopped fresh cilantro or green onions (optional)

1. Combine soy sauce, canola oil, sesame oil, ginger and hot pepper sauce in small bowl. Drain tofu and place between two paper towels. Press lightly to drain excess water from tofu. Cut tofu into 1-inch cubes. Place in shallow dish. Drizzle 2 tablespoons soy sauce mixture over tofu cubes. Set aside.

2. Combine spinach, cabbage, sugar snap peas, carrots, bean sprouts and remaining soy sauce mixture in large bowl; toss well. Top each serving with tofu mixture, peanuts and cilantro, if desired.

nutritionals

Serving Size: *about 1½ cups*, Calories: *330*, Total Fat: *20g*, Saturated Fat: *3g*, Cholesterol: *0mg*, Sodium: *1100mg*, Carbohydrate: *15g*, Dietary Fiber: *5g*, Sugar: *5g*, Protein: *23g*

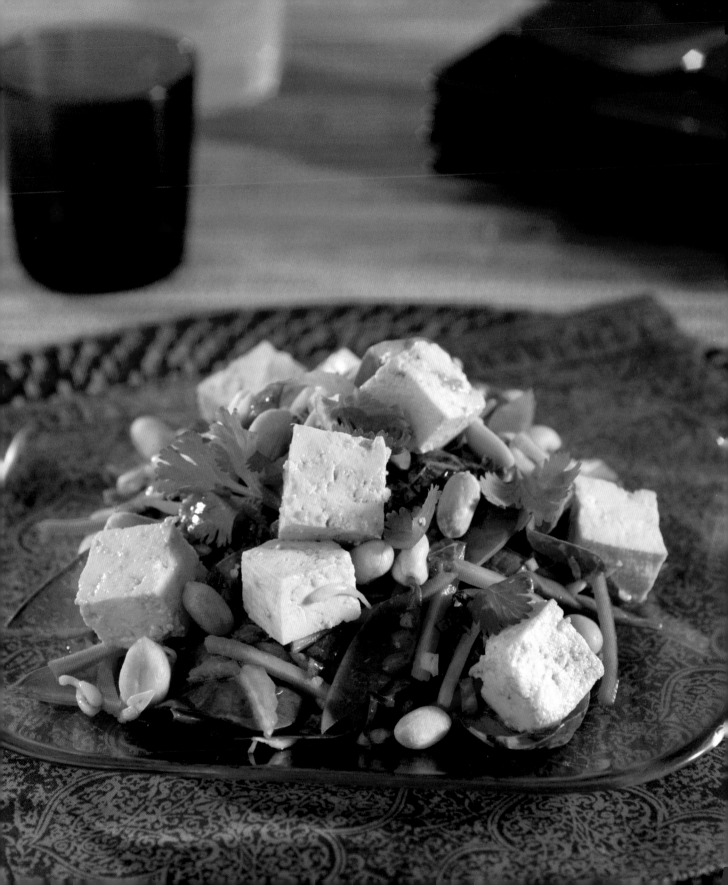

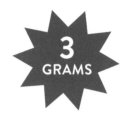

3 GRAMS

BROWN RICE, ASPARAGUS AND TOMATO SALAD

makes 4 servings

1 cup uncooked instant brown rice

12 medium spears asparagus, cooked and cut into 1-inch pieces

2 medium tomatoes

2½ teaspoons lemon juice

2 teaspoons olive oil

⅛ teaspoon salt

⅛ teaspoon black pepper

¼ cup minced fresh chives or green onions

2 teaspoons minced fresh dill

1. Bring 1 cup water to a boil in medium saucepan. Stir in rice. Bring water to a boil again. Reduce heat to low; cover and simmer 5 minutes. Remove from heat. Stir rice; cover again. Let stand 5 minutes or until water is absorbed and rice is tender. Fluff with fork; set aside.

2. Meanwhile, place asparagus in large bowl. Core tomatoes over a separate bowl to catch juice. Dice tomatoes, reserving juice. Add tomatoes to asparagus. Whisk 1½ tablespoons reserved tomato juice, lemon juice, oil, salt and pepper in small bowl until well blended. Stir in chives and dill.

3. Add rice to salad bowl. Pour in dressing; toss lightly to coat.

VARIATION: To turn this salad into a heartier main dish, add 1 cup chopped cooked chicken breast.

nutritionals

Serving Size: *about ¾ cup*, Calories: *130*, Total Fat: *4g*, Saturated Fat: *0g*, Cholesterol: *0mg*, Sodium: *80mg*, Carbohydrate: *24g*, Dietary Fiber: *3g*, Sugar: *3g*, Protein: *4g*

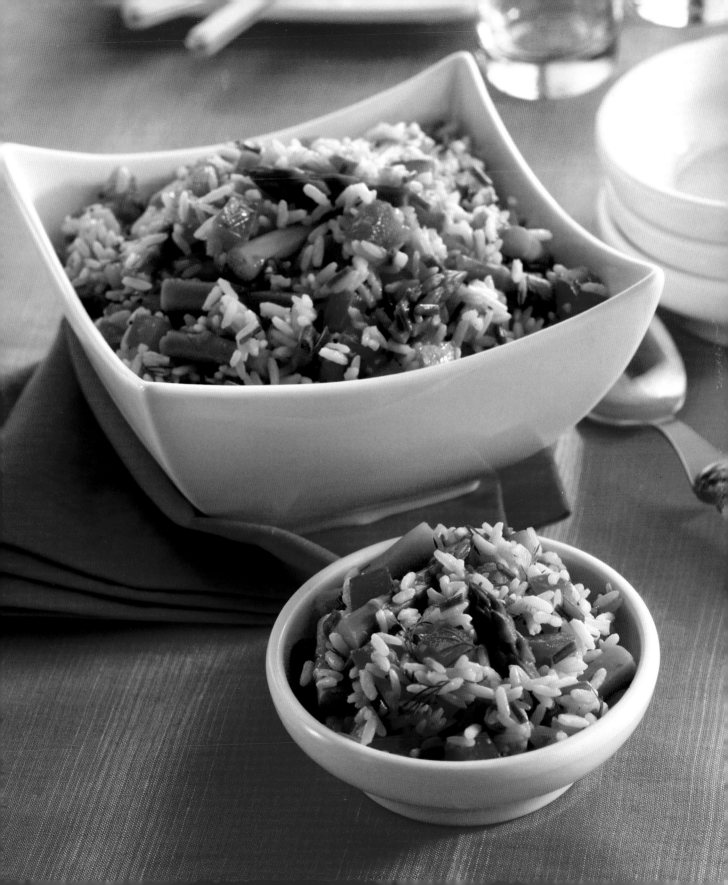

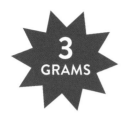

3 GRAMS

CUCUMBER-JICAMA SALAD

makes 6 servings

1 cucumber, unpeeled

1 jicama (1¼ to 1½ pounds)

½ cup thinly slivered mild red onion

2 tablespoons fresh lime juice

½ teaspoon grated lime peel

1 clove garlic, minced

¼ teaspoon salt

⅛ teaspoon crumbled dried de árbol chile or red pepper flakes

3 tablespoons vegetable oil

Leaf lettuce

Additional red onion slivers and lime wedges (optional)

1. Cut cucumber lengthwise in half; scoop out and discard seeds. Cut halves crosswise into ⅛-inch-thick slices. Peel jicama. Cut lengthwise into eight wedges; cut wedges crosswise into ⅛-inch-thick slices.

2. Combine cucumber, jicama and ½ cup onion in large bowl; toss lightly to mix. Set aside.

3. Combine lime juice, lime peel, garlic, salt and chile in small bowl. Gradually add oil, whisking continuously, until dressing is thoroughly blended.

4. Pour dressing over salad; toss lightly to coat. Cover; refrigerate 1 to 2 hours to blend flavors.

5. Serve salad in lettuce-lined salad bowl. Garnish with onion slivers and lime wedges, if desired.

TIP: To add a decorative touch to cucumber slices, score the skin of a cucumber by pulling the tines of a dinner fork along the length of the cucumber. Rotate the cucumber and repeat until completely scored. Then cut the cucumber crosswise into slices.

nutritionals

Serving Size: *about ½ cup*, Calories: *110*, Total Fat: *7g*, Saturated Fat: *1g*, Cholesterol: *0mg*, Sodium: *105mg*, Carbohydrate: *11g*, Dietary Fiber: *5g*, Sugar: *3g*, Protein: *1g*

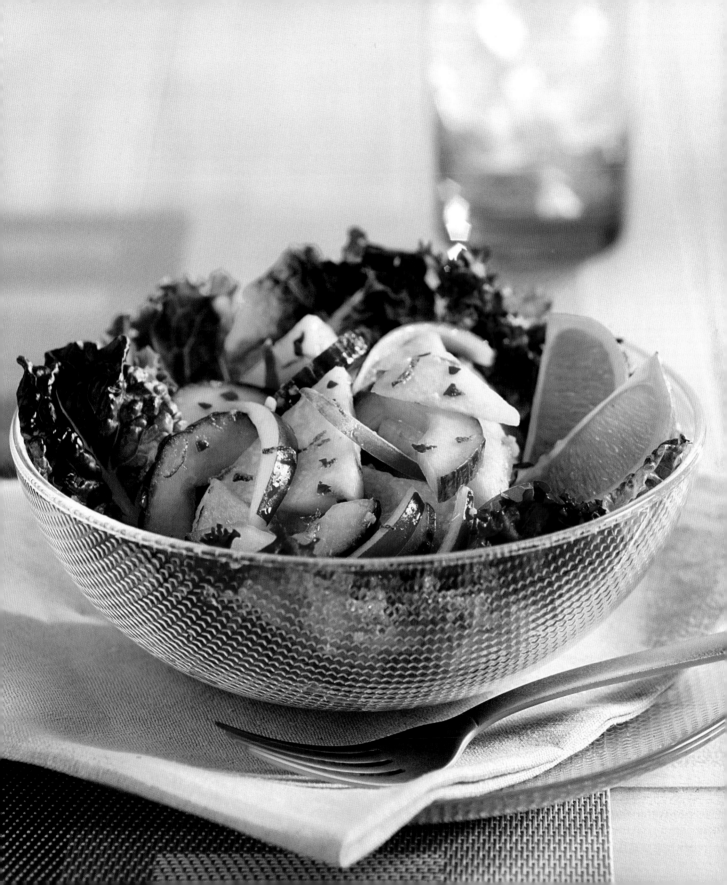

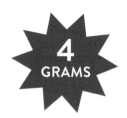

4 GRAMS

SIRLOIN STEAK WITH VEGETABLE SALAD

makes 4 servings

1   medium red bell pepper, quartered

1   medium yellow squash, halved lengthwise

1   medium onion, halved and separated

1   boneless beef top sirloin steak (about 1 pound)

1½ teaspoons steak seasoning

¼   teaspoon salt

½   cup grape tomatoes, halved

¼   cup vinaigrette salad dressing

¼   cup crumbled blue cheese

1. Spray large skillet with nonstick cooking spray; heat over medium-high heat. Add bell pepper; cook 2 to 3 minutes. Add squash and onion; cook 5 minutes on each side or until just crisp-tender. Remove vegetables and place on large cutting board.

2. Sprinkle both sides of beef with steak seasoning and salt. Add beef to skillet; cook 4 minutes on each side or to desired degree of doneness. Remove to cutting board; let stand 3 minutes before thinly slicing.

3. Meanwhile, coarsely chop vegetables and place in medium bowl.

4. Toss vegetables with tomatoes and salad dressing. Add cheese and toss gently. Serve alongside beef slices.

nutritionals

Serving Size: *3 ounces cooked beef and about ¾ cup vegetable salad*, Calories: *270*, Total Fat: *9g*, Saturated Fat: *3g*, Cholesterol: *85mg*, Sodium: *440mg*, Carbohydrate: *19g*, Dietary Fiber: *3g*, Sugar: *4g*, Protein: *29g*

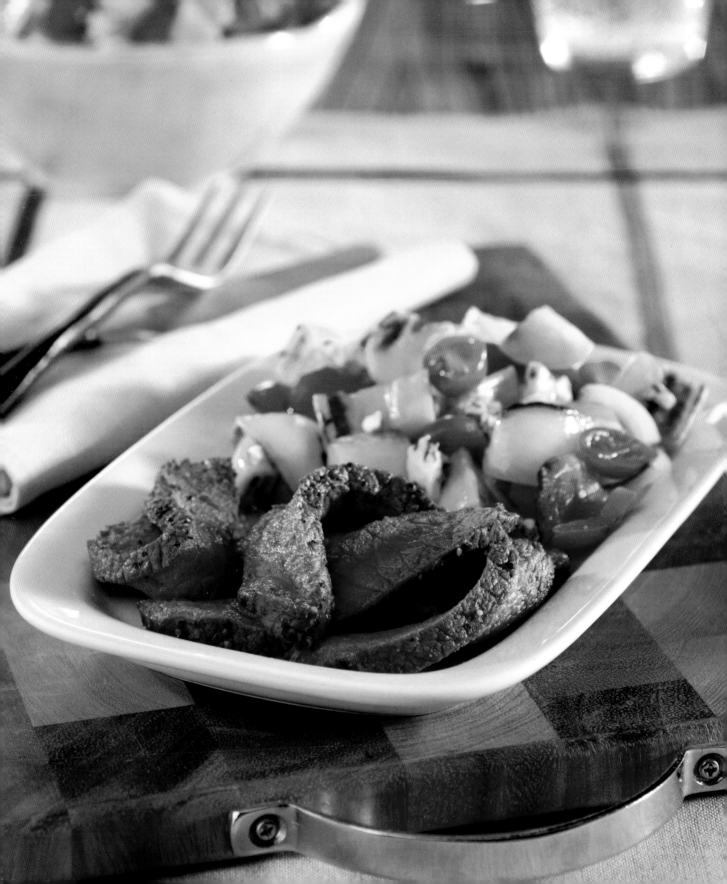

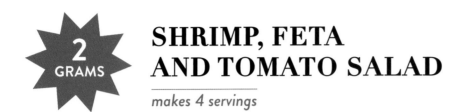

SHRIMP, FETA AND TOMATO SALAD

makes 4 servings

8 ounces cooked medium shrimp, peeled and deveined (with tails on)

1 pint (2 cups) cherry tomatoes, halved (or whole small yellow pear tomatoes)

¼ cup chopped or thinly sliced fresh basil leaves

1 tablespoon olive oil

1 tablespoon white wine vinegar

¼ teaspoon freshly ground black pepper

8 large Boston lettuce leaves

½ cup crumbled feta cheese

Combine shrimp, tomatoes, basil, oil, vinegar and pepper in medium bowl; mix well. Serve over lettuce and top with cheese.

nutritionals

Serving Size: *about ¾ cup*, Calories: *130*, Total Fat: *8g*, Saturated Fat: *3g*, Cholesterol: *80mg*, Sodium: *500mg*, Carbohydrate: *5g*, Dietary Fiber: *1g*, Sugar: *2g*, Protein: *11g*

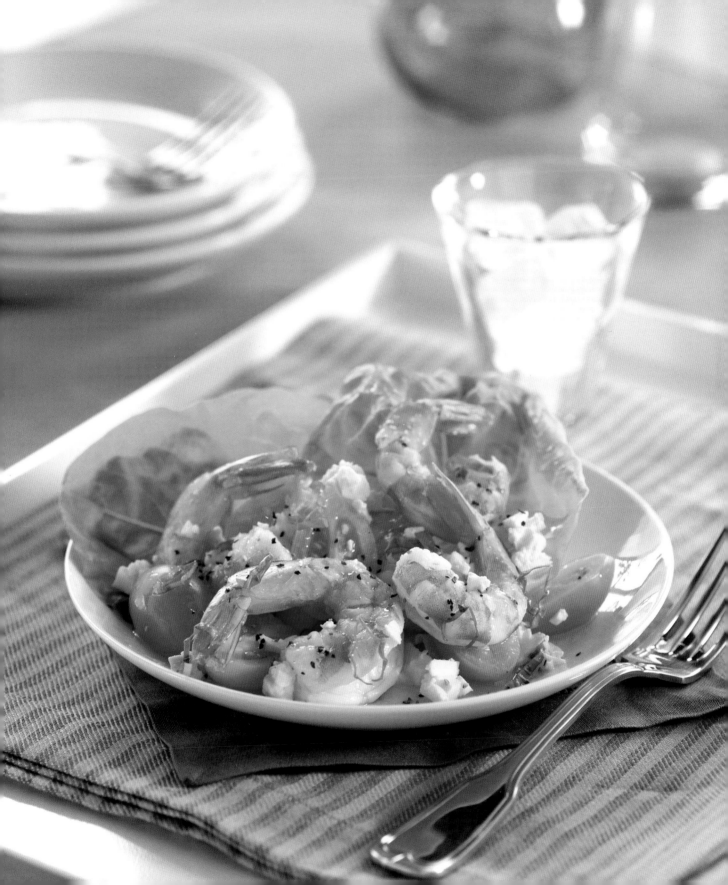

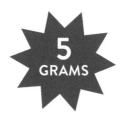
5 GRAMS

GRILLED PEACH SALAD WITH SPINACH AND RED ONION VINAIGRETTE

makes 4 servings

3 tablespoons plus
  1 teaspoon extra-virgin
  olive oil, divided

2 tablespoons rice wine
  vinegar **or** 1½ tablespoons
  balsamic vinegar

2 tablespoons finely chopped
  red onion

1 tablespoon chopped
  fresh tarragon **or** basil, **or**
  1 teaspoon dried tarragon
  or basil, crushed

  Salt and black pepper

1 cup **DOLE**® Frozen Sliced
  Peaches, partially thawed

1 package (9 ounces)
  DOLE® Spinach **or** Spring
  Mix Salad Blends

½ cup crumbled feta **or** goat
  cheese

WHISK 3 tablespoons olive oil and vinegar in small bowl. Add onion, tarragon, and season with salt and pepper.

BRUSH peach slices with remaining 1 teaspoon olive oil. Grill over a medium-hot fire or on a stovetop grill pan over medium heat, until lightly browned, about 4 to 5 minutes. Cool for 1 minute.

COMBINE spinach, peaches and cheese in large bowl. Add vinaigrette: gently toss to coat.

nutritionals

Serving Size: *¼ of recipe*, Calories: *208*, Total Fat: *16g*, Saturated Fat: *4g*, Cholesterol: *17mg*, Sodium: *893mg*, Carbohydrate: *14g*, Dietary Fiber: *4g*, Sugar: *5g*, Protein: *5g*

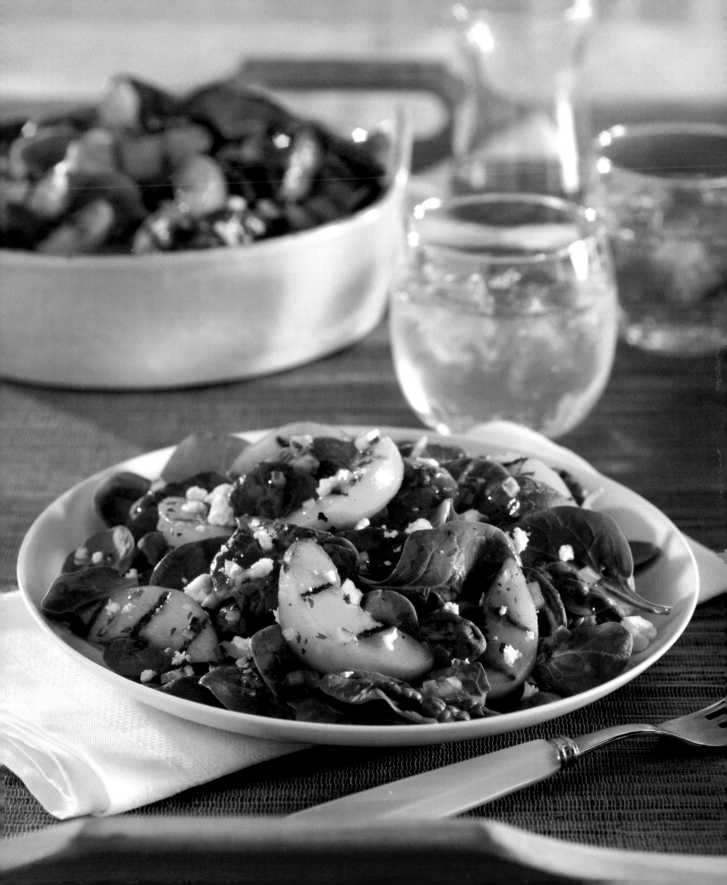

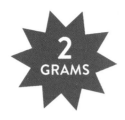

2 GRAMS

SOUTHWESTERN TUNA SALAD

makes 4 servings

2   limes, juiced, divided

12 ounces raw tuna steaks
    (about 1 inch thick)

1   pint cherry or grape
    tomatoes, halved

¼   cup diced ripe avocado
    (¼ of medium avocado)

1   jalapeño pepper,* seeded
    and minced

1   green onion, chopped
    (green part only)

1   tablespoon chopped
    fresh cilantro

1½ teaspoons canola oil

¼   teaspoon salt

¼   teaspoon ground cumin

⅛   teaspoon black pepper
    Lime wedges (optional)

**Jalapeño peppers can sting
and irritate the skin, so wear
rubber gloves when handling
peppers and do not touch
your eyes.*

1. Place juice of one lime in glass baking dish or shallow bowl. Add tuna steaks. Marinate at room temperature 30 minutes, turning once.

2. Spray stovetop grill pan with nonstick cooking spray; heat over medium heat 30 seconds. Add tuna steaks; cook 5 to 6 minutes per side. Remove and set aside until cooled to room temperature. Cut into bite-size chunks.

3. Combine tomatoes, avocado, jalapeño pepper, green onion and cilantro in large bowl. Add tuna.

4. Whisk oil, remaining lime juice, salt, cumin and black pepper in small bowl. Pour over salad; toss to coat. Garnish with lime wedges, if desired.

nutritionals

Serving Size: *about 1 cup*, Calories: *180*, Total Fat: *7g*, Saturated Fat: *2g*, Cholesterol: *30mg*, Sodium: *190mg*, Carbohydrate: *8g*, Dietary Fiber: *3g*, Sugar: *2g*, Protein: *21g*

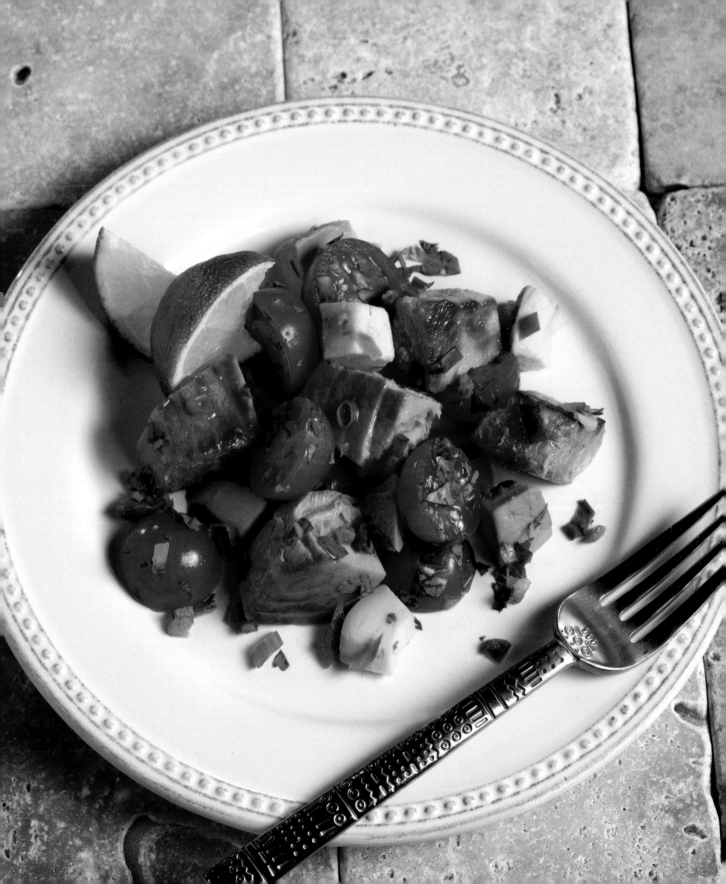

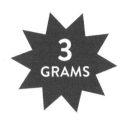
3 GRAMS

MARINATED TOMATO SALAD

makes 8 servings

1½ cups white wine or tarragon vinegar

½ teaspoon salt

¼ cup finely chopped shallots

2 tablespoons finely chopped chives

2 tablespoons fresh lemon juice

¼ teaspoon white pepper

2 tablespoons extra virgin olive oil

6 plum tomatoes, quartered

2 large yellow tomatoes,* sliced horizontally into ½-inch-thick slices

16 red cherry tomatoes, halved

16 small yellow pear tomatoes,* halved (optional)

  Sunflower sprouts (optional)

*Substitute 10 plum tomatoes, quartered, for yellow tomatoes and yellow pear tomatoes, if desired.

1. Combine vinegar and salt in large bowl; stir until salt is completely dissolved. Add shallots, chives, lemon juice and pepper; mix well. Slowly whisk in oil until well blended.

2. Add tomatoes to marinade; toss well. Cover; let stand at room temperature 30 minutes or up to 2 hours before serving.

3. To serve, divide salad equally among eight plates. Garnish with sunflower sprouts.

nutritionals

Serving Size: *about ¾ cup*, Calories: *60*, Total Fat: *4g*, Saturated Fat: *1g*, Cholesterol: *0mg*, Sodium: *160mg*, Carbohydrate: *6g*, Dietary Fiber: *2g*, Sugar: *3g*, Protein: *1g*

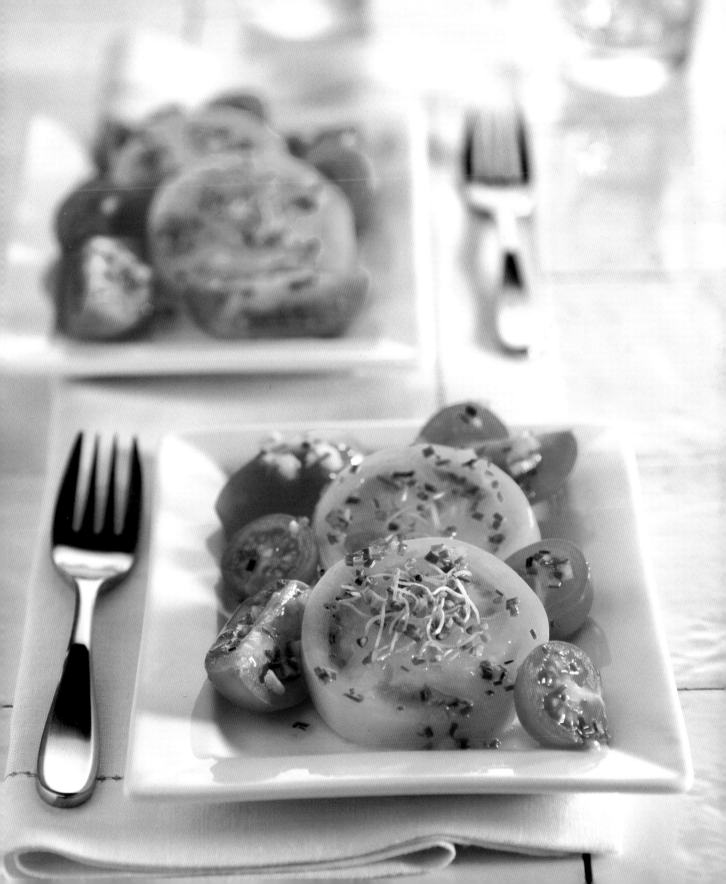

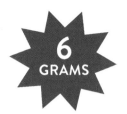

6 GRAMS

SPRINGTIME SPINACH SALAD

makes 6 side-dish servings

8 ounces fresh **DOLE®** Asparagus Spears **or** 1 package (10 ounces) frozen asparagus tips

¼ cup water

1 package (6 ounces) **DOLE®** Baby Spinach **or** Spinach and Leaf Salad Blends

1½ cups **DOLE®** Frozen Sliced Strawberries, partially thawed

½ cup julienne-sliced red onion

½ cup Raspberry Dressing (*recipe follows*) **or** red wine and vinegar dressing

⅔ cup crumbled feta **or** blue cheese

BREAK off woody ends of asparagus (the bottom 1 to 1½ inches) and discard. Cut asparagus into 1-inch lengths. Place in a microwaveable dish with water. Microwave on HIGH power for 3 minutes. Immediately rinse asparagus under cold water for 1 minute; drain well.

PLACE salad blend, drained asparagus, strawberries and onion in a large bowl.

POUR dressing over salad; toss to evenly coat. Sprinkle cheese over salad.

RASPBERRY DRESSING: Place ¾ cup thawed **DOLE®** Frozen Raspberries, ⅓ to ½ cup orange juice, ⅓ cup olive oil, 1 tablespoon honey and ¼ teaspoon salt in blender or food processor container. Cover; blend until smooth. Makes 1¼ cups.

---

nutritionals

Serving Size: *⅙ of recipe*, Calories: *140*, Total Fat: *9g*, Saturated Fat: *3g*, Cholesterol: *15mg*, Sodium: *390mg*, Carbohydrate: *13g*, Dietary Fiber: *3g*, Sugar: *6g*, Protein: *5g*

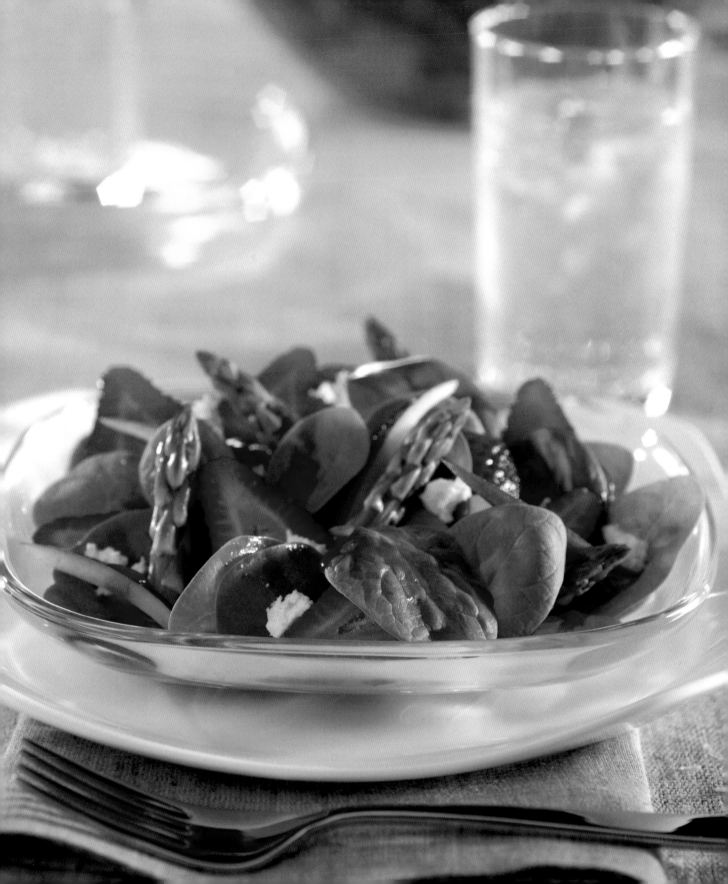

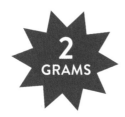

2 GRAMS

CAPRESE QUINOA SALAD

makes 6 servings

1 cup uncooked quinoa

2 cups water

½ teaspoon salt

1 container (10.5 ounces) grape tomatoes

1 package (8 ounces) fresh mozzarella pearls (small balls)

½ cup balsamic viniagrette

⅓ cup chopped fresh basil

1 clove garlic, crushed

⅛ teaspoon black pepper

1. Place quinoa in fine-mesh strainer; rinse well under cold running water.

2. Bring 2 cups water in medium saucepan to a boil over high heat; stir in quinoa and salt. Reduce heat to low. Cover; simmer 10 to 15 minutes or until quinoa is tender and water is absorbed.

3. Remove from heat; fluff and cool. Transfer to large serving bowl. Fold in tomatoes, mozzarella, viniagrette, basil, garlic and pepper.

nutritionals

Serving Size: *about ¾ cup*, Calories: *260*, Total Fat: *13g*, Saturated Fat: *6g*, Cholesterol: *25mg*, Sodium: *460mg*, Carbohydrate: *25g*, Dietary Fiber: *3g*, Sugar: *2g*, Protein: *11g*

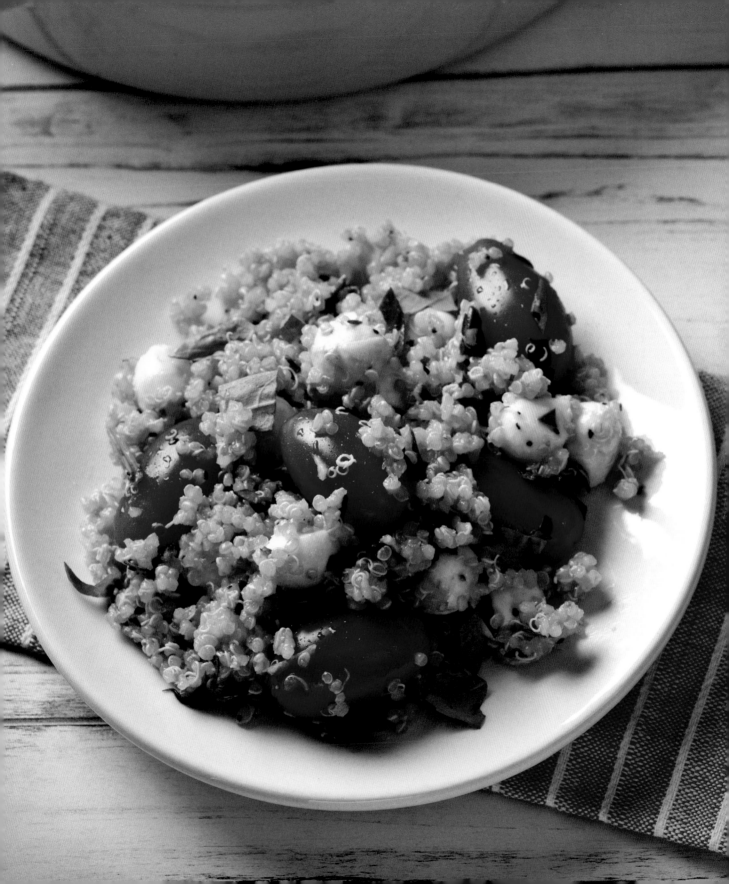

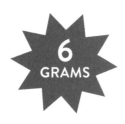

6 GRAMS

CHICKEN PEANUT SALAD

makes 6 servings

¾ cup mayonnaise

1 teaspoon ground cumin

1 teaspoon lemon juice

½ teaspoon onion powder

½ teaspoon salt

¼ teaspoon garlic powder

¼ teaspoon black pepper

3 cups diced cooked chicken

1 cup seedless grapes, cut into halves

1 cup diced jicama

½ cup chopped red bell pepper

1 large head leaf lettuce

½ cup peanuts, chopped

1. Combine mayonnaise, cumin, lemon juice, onion powder, salt, garlic powder and black pepper in small bowl; stir to blend well. Combine chicken, grapes, jicama and bell pepper in large bowl. Pour dressing over chicken mixture; stir well. Cover; refrigerate until chilled.

2. Line plates with lettuce and spoon chicken salad over top. Sprinkle with peanuts and serve immediately.

nutritionals

Serving Size: *about 1 cup*, Calories: *460*, Total Fat: *32g*, Saturated Fat: *6g*, Cholesterol: *60mg*, Sodium: *450mg*, Carbohydrate: *10g*, Dietary Fiber: *3g*, Sugar: *6g*, Protein: *39g*

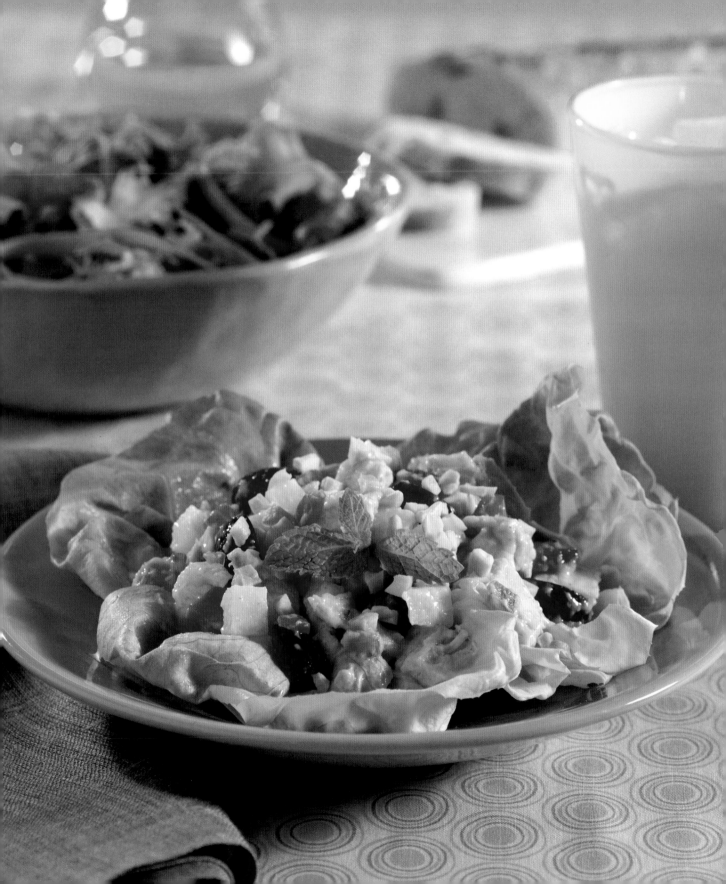

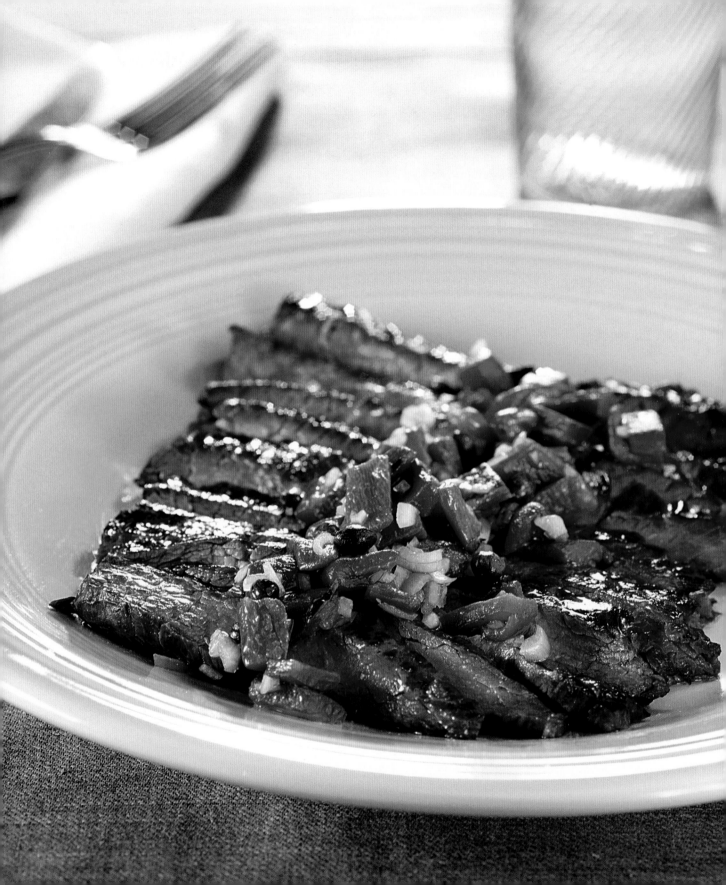

BEEF

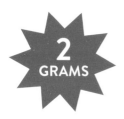
2 GRAMS

SKIRT STEAK WITH RED PEPPER CHIMICHURRI

makes 4 servings

1   pound skirt steak, trimmed

1   clove garlic, peeled and cut in half

¼   teaspoon salt

½   teaspoon black pepper, divided

1   cup diced roasted red bell pepper

1   shallot, minced

1   tablespoon capers

1½ tablespoons olive oil

1   tablespoon white wine vinegar

1   clove garlic, minced

1. Preheat broiler. Spray broiler rack with nonstick cooking spray. Rub steak on both sides with garlic clove. Season with salt and ¼ teaspoon black pepper. Place steak on broiler rack. Broil steak, 4 inches from heat, 4 to 5 minutes per side or until desired doneness.

2. To prepare chimichurri sauce, combine red bell pepper, shallot, capers, oil, vinegar, minced garlic and remaining ¼ teaspoon black pepper in small bowl.

3. To serve, thinly slice skirt steak against the grain; arrange on serving platter. Top with chimichurri sauce or serve separately.

nutritionals

Serving Size: *about 3 ounces steak and ⅓ cup sauce,* Calories: *290,* Total Fat: *19g,* Saturated Fat: *6g,* Cholesterol: *75mg,* Sodium: *510mg,* Carbohydrate: *5g,* Dietary Fiber: *1g,* Sugar: *2g,* Protein: *24g*

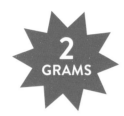

2 GRAMS

GARLIC GRILLED BEEF BROCHETTES

makes 4 servings

1 pound beef tenderloin tips or steaks, cut into 1½-inch chunks

1 small red onion, cut into ½-inch-thick wedges

1 large red or yellow bell pepper (or ½ of each), cut into 1-inch chunks

2 tablespoons chopped fresh thyme or rosemary

1. Preheat grill to medium-high heat. Alternately thread meat and vegetables onto four long bamboo or metal skewers. (If using bamboo skewers, soak in water for 20 to 30 minutes before using to prevent them from burning.)

2. Grill skewers on covered grill 5 minutes on each side. (Tenderloin will be pink in center and vegetables will be crisp-tender.) Top with thyme.

nutritionals

Serving Size: *1 skewer*, Calories: *190*, Total Fat: *9g*, Saturated Fat: *3g*, Cholesterol: *70mg*, Sodium: *50mg*, Carbohydrate: *4g*, Dietary Fiber: *1g*, Sugar: *2g*, Protein: *25g*

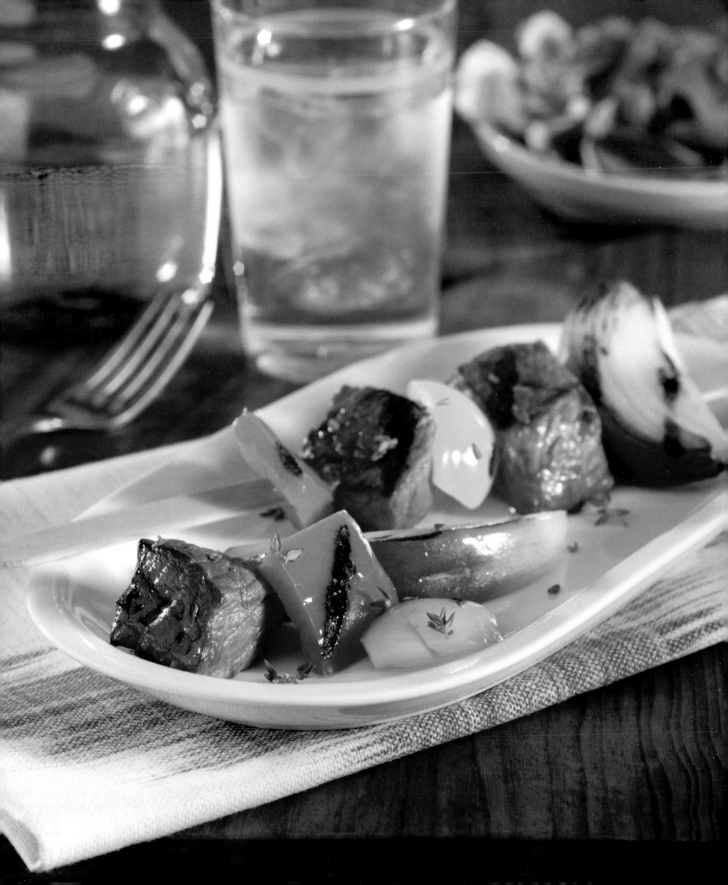

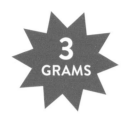
3 GRAMS

STEAK DIANE WITH CREMINI MUSHROOMS

makes 2 servings

2 beef tenderloin steaks (4 ounces each), cut ¾ inch thick

¼ teaspoon black pepper

⅓ cup sliced shallots or chopped onion

4 ounces cremini mushrooms, sliced *or* 1 (4-ounce) package sliced mixed wild mushrooms

1½ tablespoons Worcestershire sauce

1 tablespoon Dijon mustard

1. Spray large skillet with nonstick cooking spray; heat over medium-high heat. Add steaks; sprinkle with pepper. Cook 3 minutes per side for medium rare or to desired doneness. Transfer to plate; cover to keep warm.

2. Spray same skillet with cooking spray; place over medium heat. Add shallots; cook and stir 2 minutes. Add mushrooms; cook and stir 3 minutes. Add Worcestershire sauce and mustard; cook 1 minute, stirring frequently.

3. Return steaks and any accumulated juices to skillet; heat through, turning once. Transfer steaks to serving plates; top with mushroom mixture.

nutritionals

Serving Size: *about 4 ounces steak with ¼ cup mushroom mixture*, Calories: *270*, Total Fat: *10g*, Saturated Fat: *4g*, Cholesterol: *95mg*, Sodium: *390mg*, Carbohydrate: *7g*, Dietary Fiber: *1g*, Sugar: *3g*, Protein: *35g*

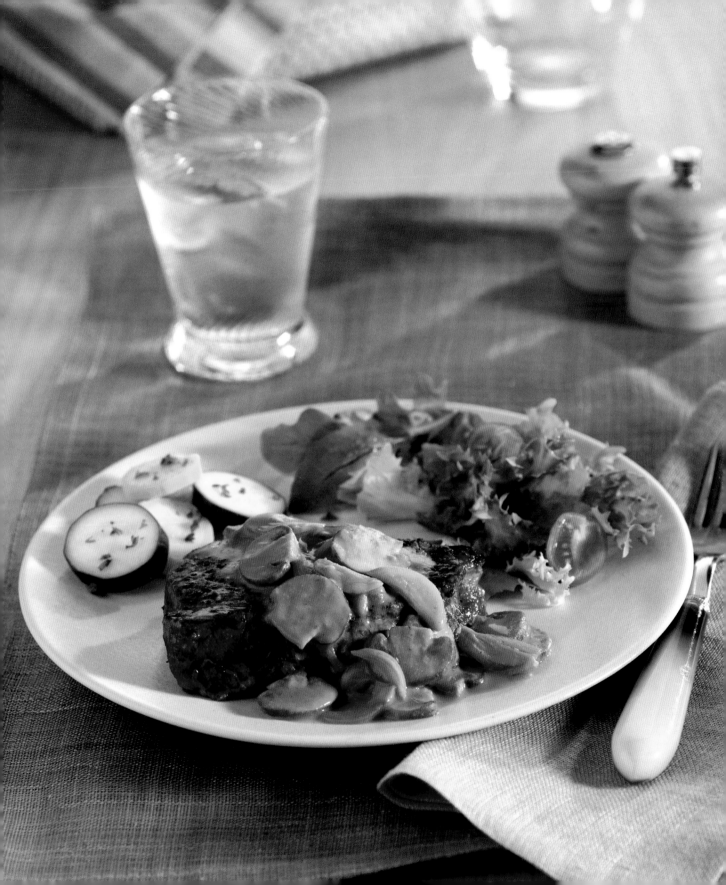

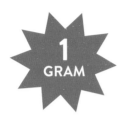

1
GRAM

BLUE CHEESE-STUFFED SIRLOIN PATTIES

makes 4 servings

1½ pounds ground beef sirloin

½ cup (2 ounces) shredded
    sharp Cheddar cheese

¼ cup crumbled blue cheese

¼ cup finely chopped fresh
    parsley

2 teaspoons Dijon mustard

1 teaspoon Worcestershire
    sauce

1 clove garlic, minced

¼ teaspoon salt

2 teaspoons olive oil

1 medium red bell pepper,
    cut into thin strips

1. Shape beef into eight patties, about 4 inches in diameter and ¼ inch thick.

2. Combine cheeses, parsley, mustard, Worcestershire sauce, garlic and ¼ teaspoon salt in small bowl; toss gently.

3. Mound one fourth of cheese mixture on each of four patties (about 3 tablespoons per patty). Top with remaining four patties; pinch edges of patties to seal completely. Set aside.

4. Heat oil in large skillet over medium-high heat. Add bell pepper; cook and stir 5 minutes or until edges of peppers begin to brown. Sprinkle with additional salt. Remove to plate; keep warm.

5. Add beef patties to same skillet; cook 5 minutes. Turn patties; top with bell peppers. Cook 4 minutes or until medium (160°F) or to desired doneness.

nutritionals

Serving Size: *1 patty with ¼ of bell peppers*, Calories: *310*, Total Fat: *17g*, Saturated Fat: *8g*, Cholesterol: *110mg*, Sodium: *500mg*, Carbohydrate: *3g*, Dietary Fiber: *1g*, Sugar: *1g*, Protein: *38g*

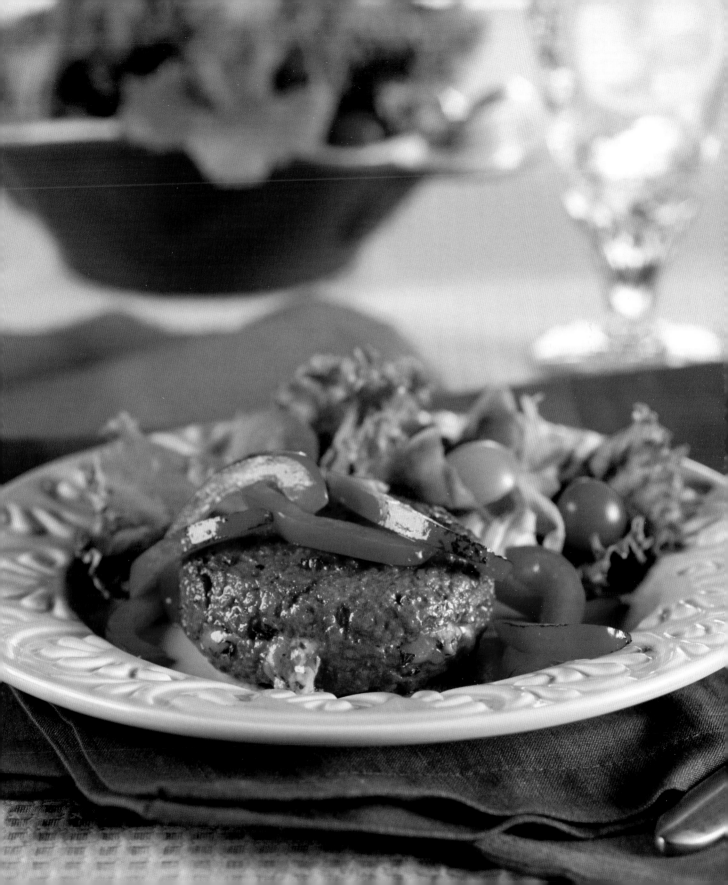

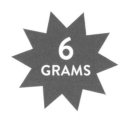
6 GRAMS

BEEF AND QUINOA STUFFED CABBAGE ROLLS

makes 4 servings

8 large green cabbage leaves, veins trimmed at bottom of each leaf

1 pound ground beef

1½ cups cooked quinoa

1 medium onion, chopped

1 cup tomato juice, divided

Salt and black pepper

SLOW COOKER DIRECTIONS

1. Heat salted water in large saucepan over high heat; bring to a boil. Add cabbage leaves; return to boil. Cook 2 minutes. Drain and let cool.

2. Combine beef, quinoa, onion, ¼ cup tomato juice, salt and pepper in large bowl; mix well. Place cabbage leaf on large work surface; top center with 2 to 3 tablespoons beef mixture. Starting at stem end, roll up jelly-roll style, folding sides in as you go. Repeat with remaining cabbage rolls and beef mixture.

3. Place cabbage rolls seam side down and side by side in single layer in slow cooker. Pour in remaining ¾ cup tomato juice. Cover; cook on LOW 5 to 6 hours.

nutritionals

Serving Size: *2 rolls*, Calories: *280*, Total Fat: *7g*, Saturated Fat: *3g*, Cholesterol: *70mg*, Sodium: *260mg*, Carbohydrate: *24g*, Dietary Fiber: *4g*, Sugar: *6g*, Protein: *29g*

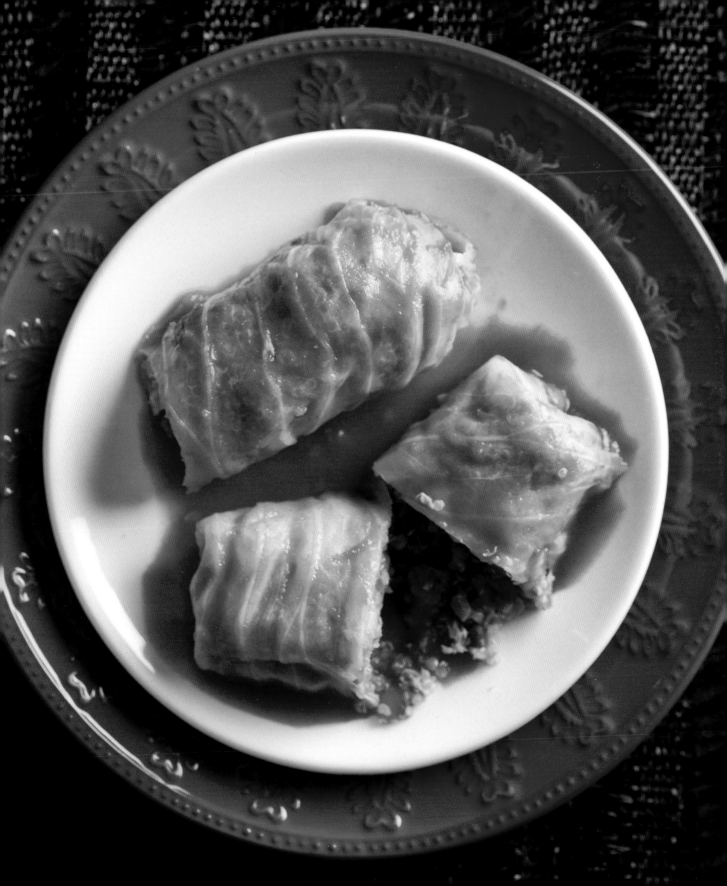

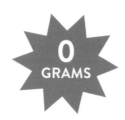
0 GRAMS

GRILLED STRIP STEAKS WITH FRESH CHIMICHURRI

makes 4 servings

4   bone-in strip steaks
     (8 ounces each),
     about 1 inch thick

¾   teaspoon salt

¾   teaspoon ground cumin

¼   teaspoon black pepper
     Chimichurri
     (recipe follows)

1. Prepare grill for direct cooking. Oil grid. Sprinkle both sides of steaks with salt, cumin and pepper.

2. Grill steaks over medium-high heat, covered, 8 to 10 minutes for medium rare or to desired doneness, turning once. Prepare and serve with Chimichurri.

CHIMICHURRI

makes about 1 cup

½   cup packed fresh basil
     leaves

⅓   cup extra virgin olive oil

¼   cup packed fresh parsley

2   tablespoons packed fresh
     cilantro

2   tablespoons fresh lemon
     juice

1   clove garlic

½   teaspoon salt

½   teaspoon grated orange
     peel

¼   teaspoon ground coriander

⅛   teaspoon black pepper

Place basil, oil, parsley, cilantro, lemon juice, garlic, salt, orange peel, coriander and pepper in food processor or blender container; purée.

nutritionals

Serving Size: *1 steak with about ¼ cup chimichurri*, Calories: *630*, Total Fat: *50g*, Saturated Fat: *15g*, Cholesterol: *165mg*, Sodium: *850mg*, Carbohydrate: *1g*, Dietary Fiber: *0g*, Sugar: *0g*, Protein: *43g*

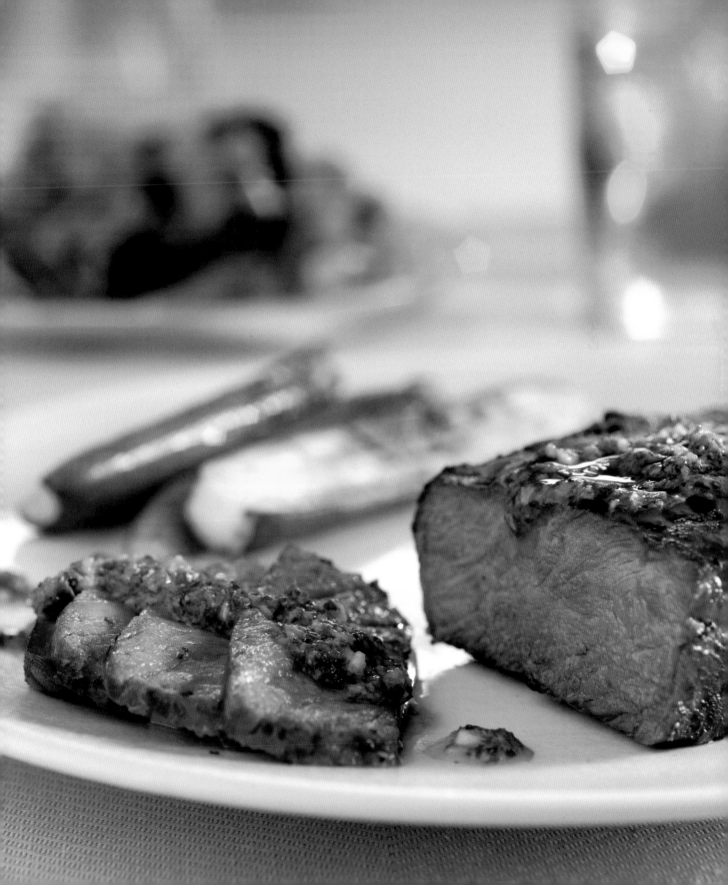

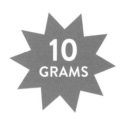

10 GRAMS

BEEF AND PINEAPPLE KABOBS

makes 4 servings

1 boneless beef top sirloin
  or top round steak (about
  1 pound)

1 small onion, finely chopped

½ cup teriyaki sauce

16 pieces (1-inch cubes) fresh
  pineapple

1 can (8 ounces) water
  chestnuts, drained

1. Cut steak into ¼-inch-thick strips. For marinade, combine onion and teriyaki sauce in small bowl. Add beef strips, stirring to coat.

2. Alternately thread beef strips (weaving back and forth), pineapple cubes and water chestnuts onto four bamboo or thin metal skewers. (If using bamboo skewers, soak in water for 20 to 30 minutes before using to prevent them from burning.)

3. Place kabobs on grid over medium coals. Grill 4 minutes, turning once, or until meat is cooked through. Serve immediately.

NOTE: Recipe can also be prepared with flank steak.

SERVING SUGGESTION: Serve with stir-fried broccoli, mushrooms and red bell peppers.

---

nutritionals

Serving Size: *1 kabob*, Calories: *210*, Total Fat: *5g*, Saturated Fat: *2g*, Cholesterol: *60mg*, Sodium: *1270mg*, Carbohydrate: *16g*, Dietary Fiber: *2g*, Sugar: *10g*, Protein: *25g*

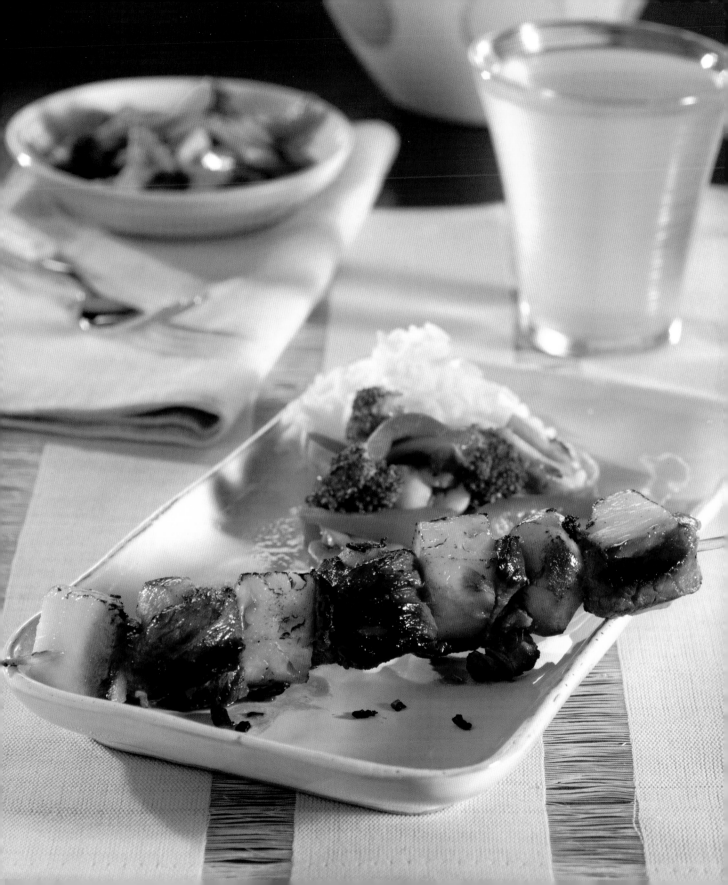

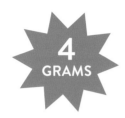

4 GRAMS

BRISKET WITH BACON, BLUE CHEESE AND ONIONS

makes 10 servings

2 large sweet onions,* sliced into ½-inch rounds

6 slices bacon, divided

1 flat-cut boneless beef brisket (about 3½ pounds)

Salt and black pepper

2 cans (10½ ounces each) condensed beef consommé, undiluted

1 teaspoon cracked black peppercorns

¾ cup crumbled blue cheese

*Maui, Vidalia or Walla Walla onions are preferred.

SLOW COOKER DIRECTIONS

1. Coat 5- to 6-quart slow cooker with nonstick cooking spray. Line bottom with onion slices.

2. Heat large skillet over medium-high heat. Add bacon; cook until chewy, not crisp. Drain on paper towel-lined plate. Reserve drippings in skillet. Chop bacon.

3. Season brisket with salt and pepper. Sear brisket in bacon drippings on all sides. Remove to slow cooker.

4. Pour consommé into slow cooker. Sprinkle with peppercorns and half of bacon. Cover; cook on HIGH 5 to 7 hours.

5. Remove brisket to large cutting board; cover with foil. Let stand 10 to 15 minutes. Slice against the grain into ¾-inch slices.

6. To serve, arrange brisket slices on plates; top with onions, blue cheese and remaining bacon. Season cooking liquid with salt or pepper and serve with brisket.

---

nutritionals

Serving Size: *about 4½ ounces brisket with ½ cup onion mixture*, Calories: *470*, Total Fat: *29g*, Saturated Fat: *12g*, Cholesterol: *155mg*, Sodium: *650mg*, Carbohydrate: *6g*, Dietary Fiber: *1g*, Sugar: *4g*, Protein: *45g*

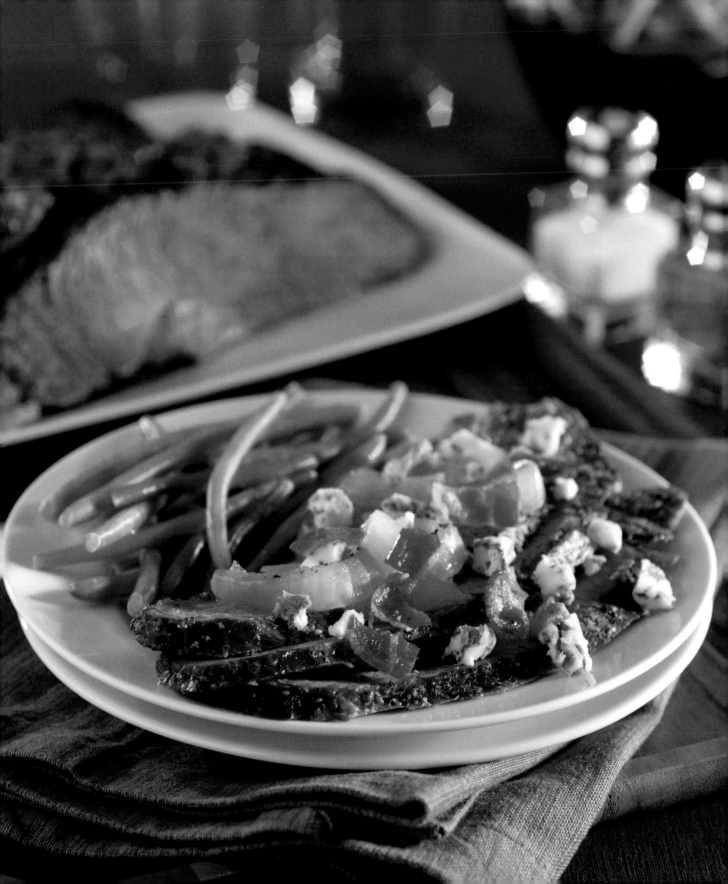

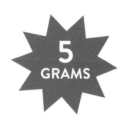

5 GRAMS

GREEK-STYLE BEEF KABOBS

makes 4 servings

1 pound boneless beef top sirloin steak (1 inch thick), cut into 16 pieces

¼ cup Italian salad dressing

3 tablespoons fresh lemon juice, divided

1 tablespoon dried oregano

1 tablespoon Worcestershire sauce

2 teaspoons dried basil

1 teaspoon grated lemon peel

⅛ teaspoon red pepper flakes

1 large green bell pepper, cut into 16 pieces

16 cherry tomatoes

2 teaspoons olive oil

⅛ teaspoon salt

1. Combine beef, salad dressing, 2 tablespoons lemon juice, oregano, Worcestershire sauce, basil, lemon peel and red pepper flakes in large resealable food storage bag. Seal bag; turn to coat. Marinate in refrigerator at least 8 hours or overnight, turning occasionally.

2. Preheat broiler. Remove beef from marinade; reserve marinade. Thread four 10-inch metal skewers with beef, alternating with bell pepper and tomatoes. Spray rimmed baking sheet or broiler pan with nonstick cooking spray. Brush kabobs with marinade; place on baking sheet. Discard remaining marinade. Broil kabobs 3 minutes. Turn over; broil 2 minutes or until desired doneness is reached. *Do not overcook.* Remove skewers to serving platter.

3. Add remaining 1 tablespoon lemon juice, oil and salt to pan drippings on baking sheet; stir well, scraping bottom of pan with flat spatula. Pour juices over kabobs.

nutritionals

Serving Size: *1 kabob*, Calories: *280*, Total Fat: *12g*, Saturated Fat: *4g*, Cholesterol: *90mg*, Sodium: *340mg*, Carbohydrate: *8g*, Dietary Fiber: *2g*, Sugar: *5g*, Protein: *35g*

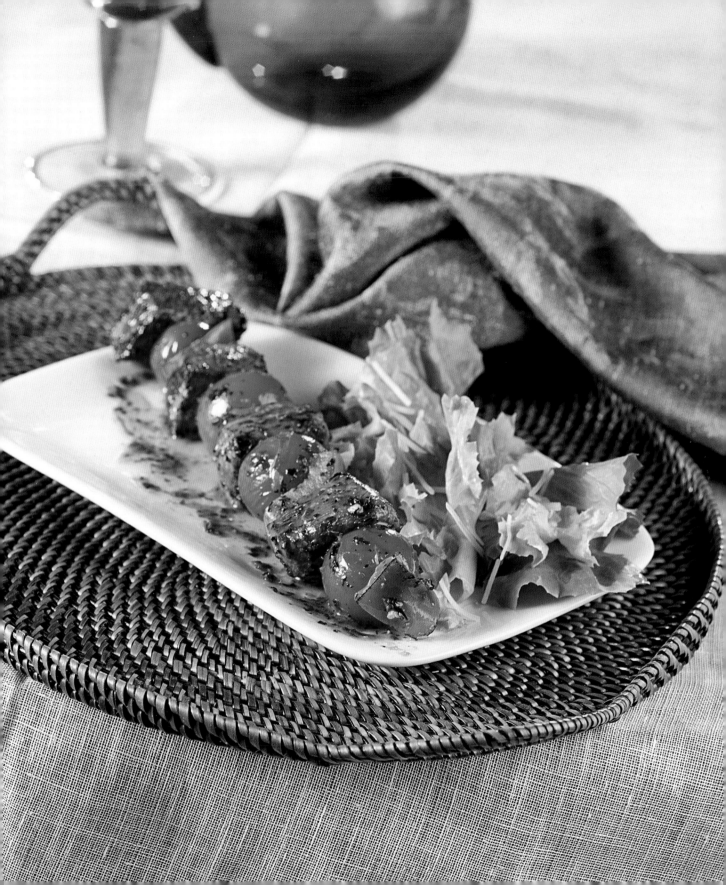

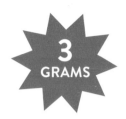

3 GRAMS

MINI ROASTED RED PEPPER MEAT LOAVES

makes 4 servings

1 jar (16 ounces) roasted red peppers

1½ pounds 90% lean ground beef

4 eggs

1 teaspoon salt

½ teaspoon Italian seasoning

¼ teaspoon black pepper

1. Preheat oven to 350°F.

2. Drain red peppers; discard juice. Thinly slice half of peppers; set aside. Finely dice remaining peppers; place in large bowl. Add beef, eggs, salt, Italian seasoning and black pepper; mix well.

3. Press mixture evenly into four miniature nonstick loaf pans. Arrange sliced red peppers over top; press lightly into meat.

4. Bake 30 minutes or until loaves are cooked through (160°F). Carefully drain juices from edges of pans. Let stand in pans 5 minutes. Cut into slices.

nutritionals

Serving Size: *1 loaf*, Calories: *410*, Total Fat: *22g*, Saturated Fat: *8g*, Cholesterol: *295mg*, Sodium: *890mg*, Carbohydrate: *6g*, Dietary Fiber: *1g*, Sugar: *3g*, Protein: *42g*

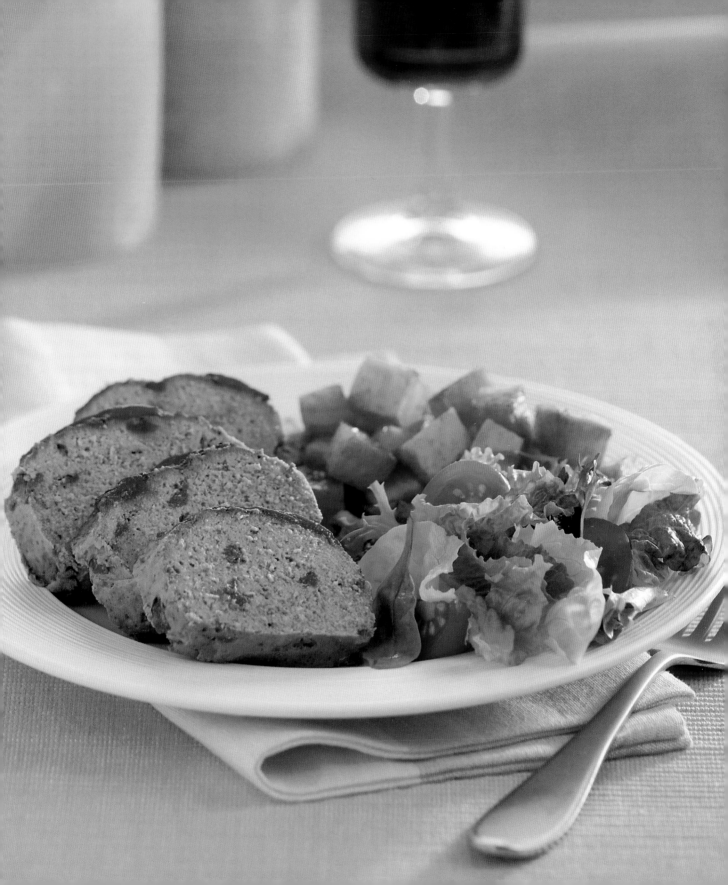

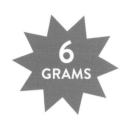

6 GRAMS

ALMOST STUFFED PEPPERS

makes 4 servings

12 ounces 90% lean ground beef

1 package (1 ounce) taco seasoning mix

1 can (about 14 ounces) diced tomatoes

½ (about 15-ounce) can black beans, rinsed and drained

½ cup finely chopped green onions (white and green parts)

2 medium or large green bell peppers, halved vertically (stems and seeds removed)

¼ cup sour cream

2 tablespoons chopped fresh cilantro

1. Spray large skillet with nonstick cooking spray; heat over medium-high heat. Add beef; cook and stir 6 to 8 minutes or until browned. Drain fat. Add taco seasoning mix, tomatoes, beans and green onions; stir until well blended. Top with bell pepper halves, cut side down. Reduce heat to low. Cover; simmer 30 minutes or until bell peppers are just tender when pierced with a fork.

2. Place one bell pepper half on each of four dinner plates, spoon equal amounts of beef mixture in each half (it will overflow), spoon 1 tablespoon sour cream on top of each and sprinkle evenly with cilantro.

nutritionals

Serving Size: *1 pepper half and 1 cup filling*, Calories: *290*, Total Fat: *12g*, Saturated Fat: *5g*, Cholesterol: *60mg*, Sodium: *980mg*, Carbohydrate: *21g*, Dietary Fiber: *5g*, Sugar: *6g*, Protein: *21g*

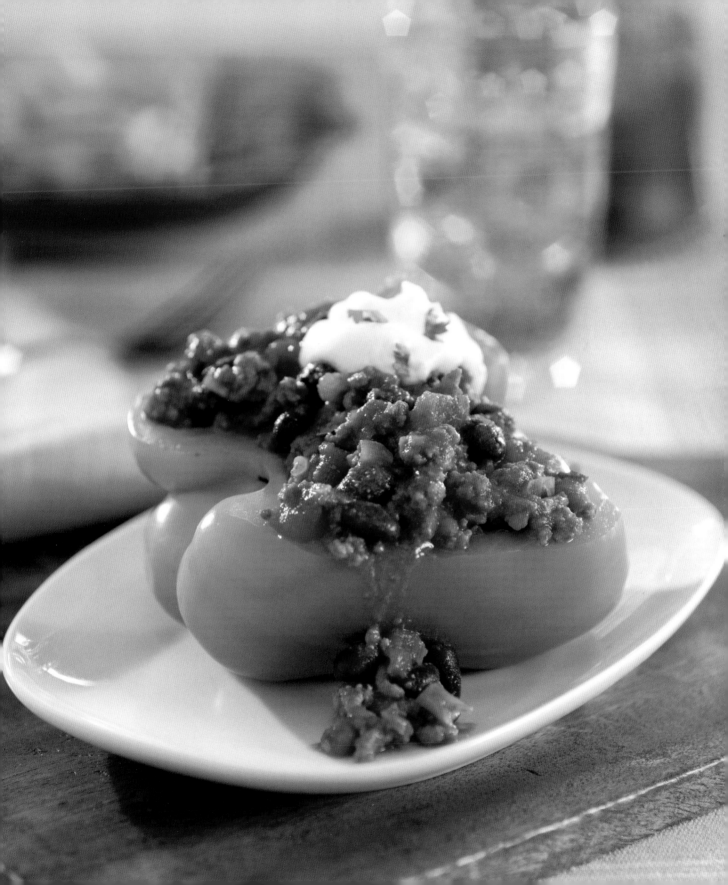

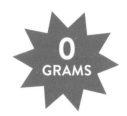

0 GRAMS

BEEF TENDERLOIN WITH HIGH SPICE RUB

makes 8 servings

1   tablespoon onion powder

2   teaspoons dried thyme

1   teaspoon ground cumin

1   teaspoon black pepper or lemon-pepper seasoning

¾   teaspoon ground allspice

½   teaspoon salt

⅛   teaspoon ground red pepper

2   pounds boneless beef tenderloin

¼   cup water

1. Combine onion powder, thyme, cumin, black pepper, allspice, salt and red pepper in small bowl; stir to blend. Sprinkle evenly over all sides of beef. Press down firmly to allow seasonings to adhere. Wrap tightly in plastic wrap; refrigerate 24 hours.

2. Preheat oven to 400°F. Coat large skillet with nonstick cooking spray; heat over medium-high heat. Add beef; cook 3 minutes. Turn; cook 2 minutes or until richly browned. Using a flat spatula, transfer beef to a rimmed baking pan coated with cooking spray. Add water to pan residue and cook 15 seconds, scraping bottom of skillet. Drizzle over beef.

3. Bake, uncovered, 25 minutes or until meat thermometer registers 135°F or desired degree of doneness. Remove from oven, cover tightly with foil and let stand 10 minutes.

4. Place beef on large cutting board, slice and arrange on serving platter. If desired, stir and spoon pan drippings evenly over all.

TIP: Pair this recipe with leafy green vegetables, such as broccoli rabe, for a complete and nutritious meal.

nutritionals

Serving Size: *about 3 ounces beef*, Calories: *180*, Total Fat: *8g*, Saturated Fat: *3g*, Cholesterol: *70mg*, Sodium: *200mg*, Carbohydrate: *1g*, Dietary Fiber: *0g*, Sugar: *0g*, Protein: *25g*

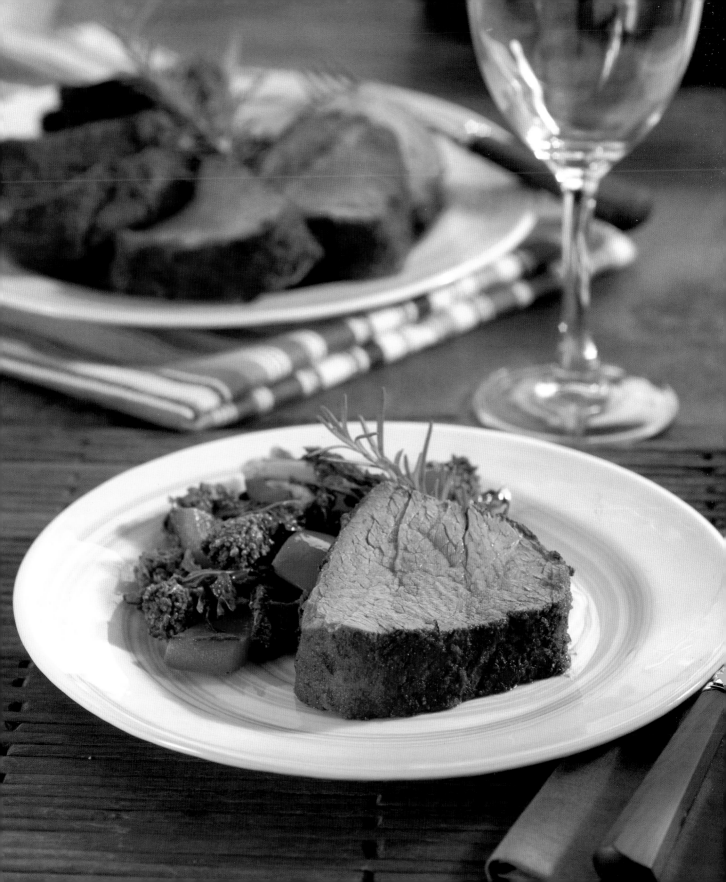

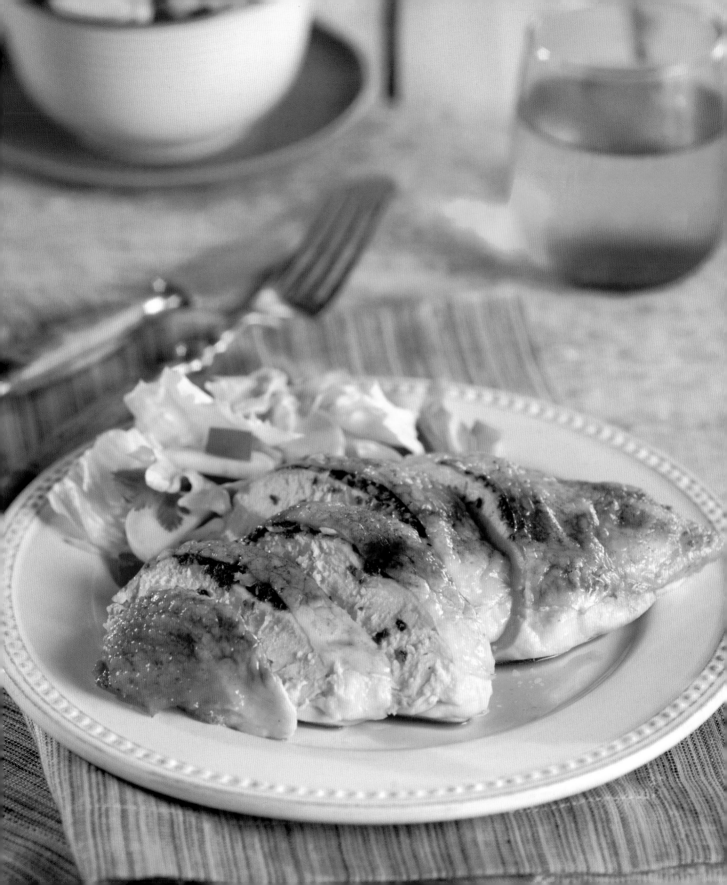

POULTRY

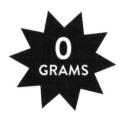

0 GRAMS

CILANTRO-STUFFED CHICKEN BREASTS

makes 4 servings

2 cloves garlic

1 cup packed fresh cilantro leaves

1 tablespoon plus 2 teaspoons soy sauce, divided

1 tablespoon peanut or vegetable oil

4 boneless chicken breasts (about 1¼ pounds)

1 tablespoon dark sesame oil

1. Preheat oven to 350°F. Mince garlic in blender or food processor. Add cilantro; process until cilantro is minced. Add 2 teaspoons soy sauce and peanut oil; process until paste forms.

2. With rubber spatula or fingers, distribute about 1 tablespoon cilantro mixture evenly under skin of each chicken breast, taking care not to puncture skin.

3. Place chicken on rack in shallow, foil-lined baking pan. Combine remaining 1 tablespoon soy sauce and sesame oil in small bowl. Brush half of mixture evenly over chicken. Bake 25 minutes; brush remaining soy sauce mixture evenly over chicken. Bake 10 minutes or until juices run clear.

nutritionals

Serving Size: *1 chicken breast*, Calories: *180*, Total Fat: *9g*, Saturated Fat: *2g*, Cholesterol: *65mg*, Sodium: *530mg*, Carbohydrate: *1g*, Dietary Fiber: *0g*, Sugar: *0g*, Protein: *21g*

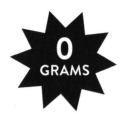

0 GRAMS

SPICY TURKEY WITH CITRUS AU JUS

makes 6 servings

1 bone-in turkey breast (about 4 pounds)

¼ cup (½ stick) butter, softened

Grated peel of 1 lemon

1 teaspoon chili powder

¼ to ½ teaspoon black pepper

⅛ to ¼ teaspoon red pepper flakes

1 tablespoon lemon juice

SLOW COOKER DIRECTIONS

1. Lightly coat slow cooker with nonstick cooking spray. Add turkey breast.

2. Mix butter, lemon peel, chili powder, black pepper and red pepper flakes in small bowl until well blended. Spread mixture over top and sides of turkey. Cover; cook on LOW 4 to 5 hours or on HIGH 2½ to 3 hours or until meat thermometer reaches 165°F.

3. Remove turkey to large cutting board. Cover loosely with foil; let stand 10 to 15 minutes.

4. Stir lemon juice into cooking liquid. Strain; discard solids. Let mixture stand 15 minutes. Skim and discard excess fat. Serve au jus with turkey.

nutritionals

Serving Size: *4 ounces*, Calories: *230*, Total Fat: *15g*, Saturated Fat: *7g*, Cholesterol: *85mg*, Sodium: *135mg*, Carbohydrate: *1g*, Dietary Fiber: *0g*, Sugar: *0g*, Protein: *23g*

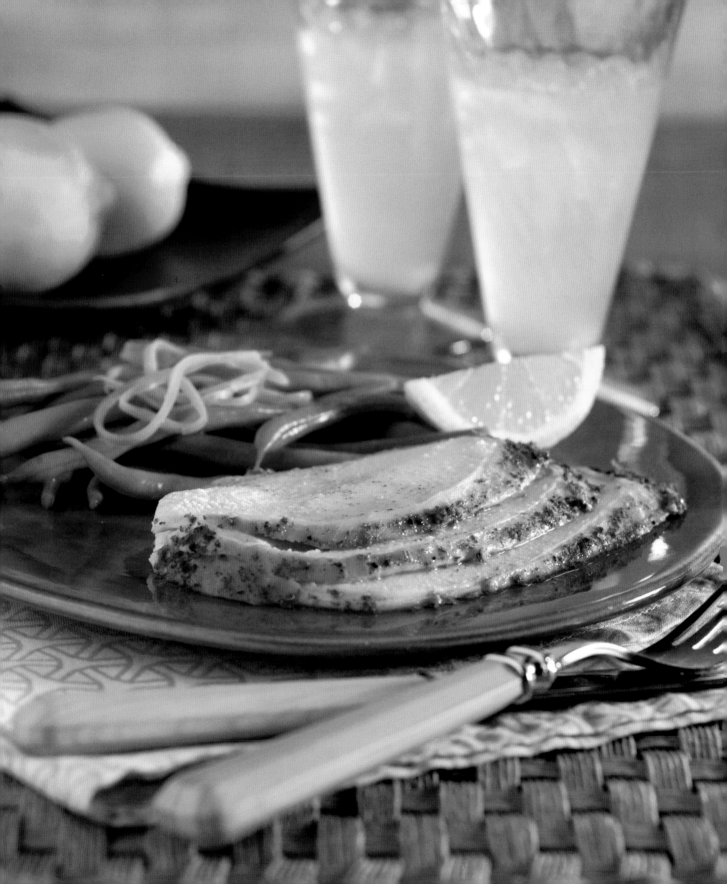

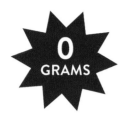

0 GRAMS

GRILLED CHICKEN WITH CHIMICHURRI SALSA

makes 4 servings

4 boneless skinless chicken breasts (6 ounces each)

½ cup plus 4 teaspoons olive oil, divided

Salt and black pepper

½ cup finely chopped fresh parsley

¼ cup white wine vinegar

2 tablespoons finely chopped onion

3 cloves garlic, minced

1 fresh or canned jalapeño pepper,* finely chopped

2 teaspoons dried oregano

Jalapeño peppers can sting and irritate the skin, so wear rubber gloves when handling peppers and do not touch your eyes.

1. Prepare grill for direct cooking.

2. Brush chicken with 4 teaspoons oil; season with salt and black pepper. Place on grid over medium heat. Grill, covered, 10 to 16 minutes or until chicken is no longer pink in center, turning once.

3. For salsa, combine parsley, remaining ½ cup oil, vinegar, onion, garlic, jalapeño pepper and oregano in small bowl. Season with salt and black pepper. Serve over chicken.

TIP: Chimichurri salsa has a fresh, green color. Serve it with grilled steak or fish as well as chicken. Chimichurri will remain fresh tasting for 24 hours.

---

nutritionals

Serving Size: *1 chicken breast with ¼ of salsa*, Calories: *500*, Total Fat: *37g*, Saturated Fat: *6g*, Cholesterol: *125mg*, Sodium: *80mg*, Carbohydrate: *3g*, Dietary Fiber: *1g*, Sugar: *0g*, Protein: *39g*

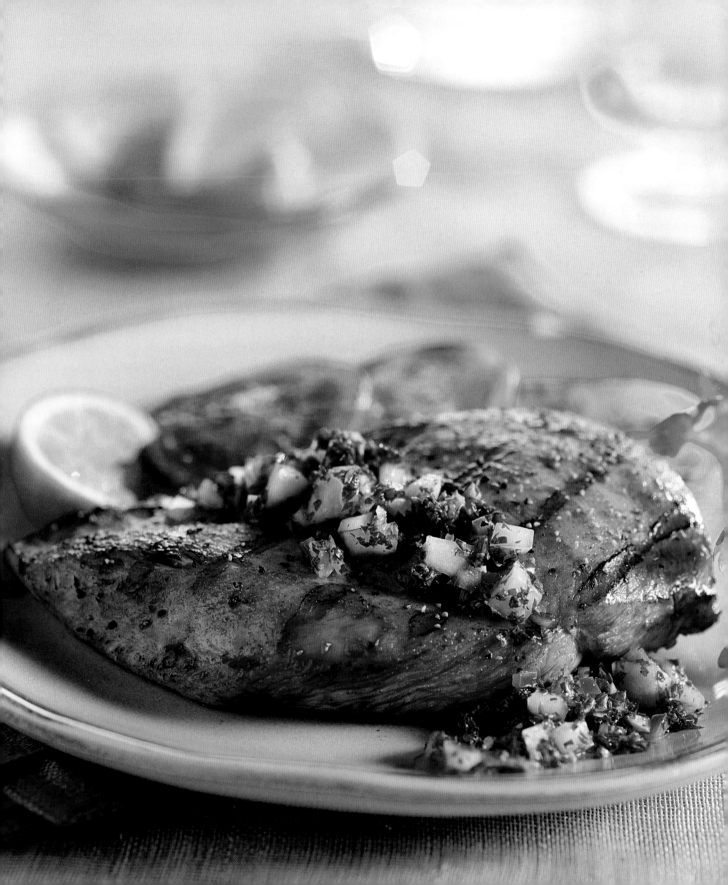

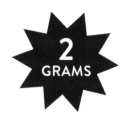

2 GRAMS

TUSCAN TURKEY AND WHITE BEAN SKILLET

makes 6 servings

1   teaspoon dried rosemary, divided

½   teaspoon garlic salt

½   teaspoon black pepper, divided

1   pound turkey breast cutlets, pounded to ¼-inch thickness

2   teaspoons canola oil

1   can (about 15 ounces) navy beans or Great Northern beans, rinsed and drained

1   can (about 14 ounces) fire-roasted diced tomatoes

¼   cup grated Parmesan cheese

1. Combine ½ teaspoon rosemary, garlic salt and ¼ teaspoon pepper in small bowl; mix well. Sprinkle over turkey.

2. Heat 1 teaspoon oil in large skillet over medium heat. Add half of turkey; cook 2 to 3 minutes per side or until no longer pink in center. Remove to platter; tent with foil to keep warm. Repeat with remaining 1 teaspoon oil and turkey.

3. Add beans, tomatoes, remaining ½ teaspoon rosemary and ¼ teaspoon pepper to skillet; bring to a boil over high heat. Reduce heat to low; simmer 5 minutes.

4. Spoon bean mixture over turkey; sprinkle with cheese.

nutritionals

Serving Size: *4 ounces*, Calories: *210*, Total Fat: *4g*, Saturated Fat: *1g*, Cholesterol: *30mg*, Sodium: *690mg*, Carbohydrate: *18g*, Dietary Fiber: *4g*, Sugar: *2g*, Protein: *27g*

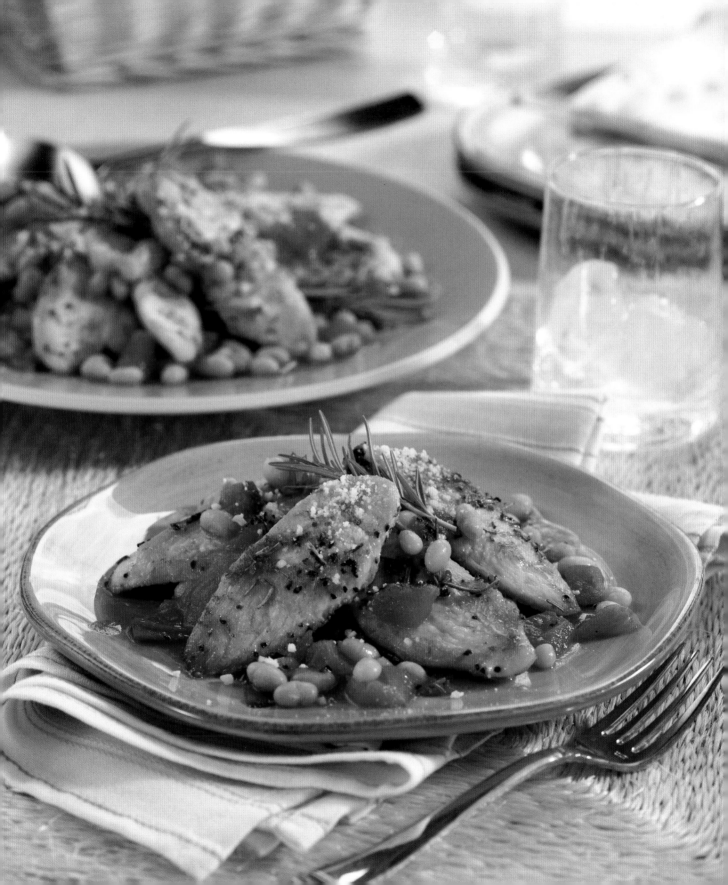

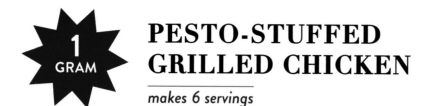

PESTO-STUFFED GRILLED CHICKEN

makes 6 servings

1 fresh or thawed frozen roasting chicken or capon (6 to 7 pounds)

½ cup prepared pesto

2 tablespoons extra virgin olive oil

2 tablespoons fresh lemon juice

Fresh basil leaves and red onion slices (optional)

1. Prepare grill with foil drip pan. Bank briquettes on either side of drip pan for indirect cooking.

2. Remove giblets from chicken cavity; reserve for another use. Loosen skin over breast of chicken by pushing fingers between skin and meat, taking care not to tear skin. Do not loosen skin over wings and drumsticks. Using rubber spatula or small spoon, spread pesto under breast skin; massage skin to evenly spread pesto. Combine oil and lemon juice in small bowl; brush over chicken skin. Insert meat thermometer into center of thickest part of thigh, not touching bone. Tuck wings under back; tie legs together with kitchen string.

3. Place chicken, breast side up, on grid directly over drip pan. Grill, covered, over medium-low coals 1 hour 10 minutes to 1 hour 30 minutes or until thermometer registers 185°F, adding 4 to 9 briquettes to both sides of fire after 45 minutes to maintain medium-low coals. Transfer chicken to large cutting board; tent with foil. Let stand 15 minutes before carving. Garnish with basil and red onion.

---

nutritionals

Serving Size: *4 ounces*, Calories: *280*, Total Fat: *18g*, Saturated Fat: *4g*, Cholesterol: *80mg*, Sodium: *410mg*, Carbohydrate: *4g*, Dietary Fiber: *0g*, Sugar: *1g*, Protein: *25g*

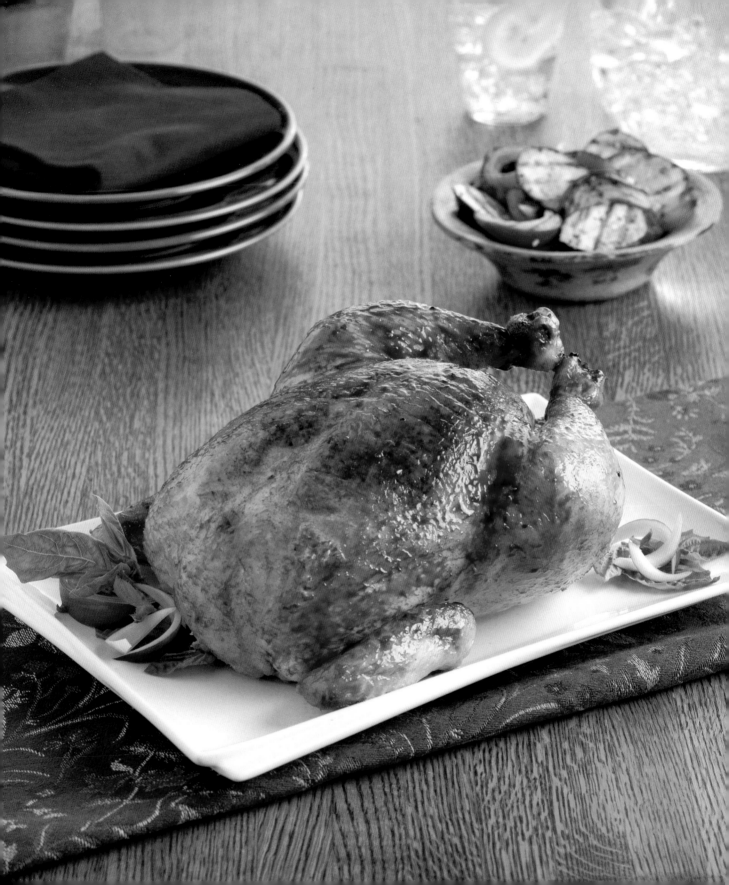

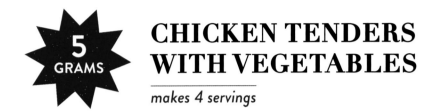

CHICKEN TENDERS WITH VEGETABLES

makes 4 servings

8 ounces chicken tenders (about ½ pound)

2 teaspoons Italian seasoning

¼ teaspoon salt

¼ teaspoon black pepper

3 teaspoons olive oil, divided

¾ cup chopped yellow onion

¾ cup finely diced carrots (about 3 medium)

½ cup finely diced celery (2 medium)

1 can (about 14 ounces) diced tomatoes, undrained

1 clove garlic, minced

1. Sprinkle chicken with Italian seasoning, salt and pepper. Heat 2 teaspoons oil in large skillet over medium-high heat. Add chicken; cook 6 minutes or until browned on both sides and chicken is no longer pink in center. Remove chicken from skillet; cover to keep warm.

2. Reduce heat to medium. Add remaining 1 teaspoon oil to skillet. Add onion, carrots and celery; cook and stir 5 minutes or until vegetables begin to soften.

3. Return chicken to skillet. Add tomatoes with juice and garlic; stir to blend. Reduce heat to low. Cover; simmer 10 minutes or until vegetables are heated through.

NOTE: Chicken "tenders" or "supremes" are the lean, tender strips that are found on the underside of the breast. They are skinless and boneless and have virtually no waste.

nutritionals

Serving Size: *3 ounces chicken and ⅔ cup vegetables*, Calories: *230*, Total Fat: *13g*, Saturated Fat: *3g*, Cholesterol: *25mg*, Sodium: *710mg*, Carbohydrate: *19g*, Dietary Fiber: *3g*, Sugar: *5g*, Protein: *10g*

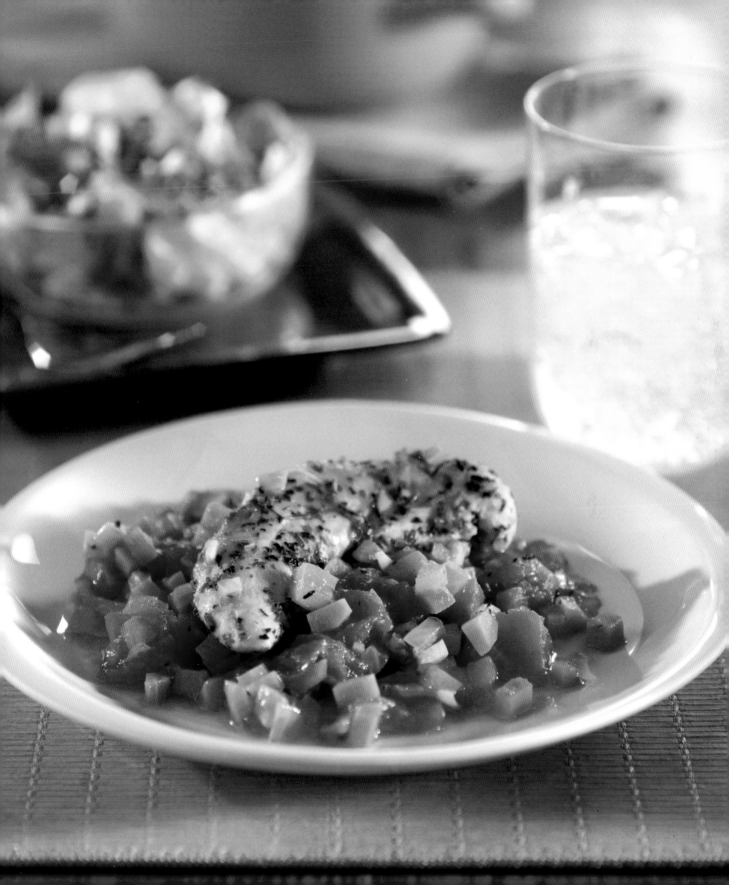

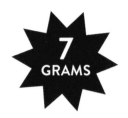

7 GRAMS

BROILED TURKEY TENDERLOIN KABOBS

makes 4 servings

¼ cup orange juice

2 tablespoons soy sauce, divided

1 clove garlic, minced

1 teaspoon fresh grated ginger

12 ounces turkey tenderloin (about 2 medium), cut into 1-inch cubes

1 green bell pepper, cut into 1-inch pieces

1 red onion, cut into 1½-inch pieces

1 cup hot cooked brown rice

1. Combine orange juice, 1 tablespoon soy sauce, garlic and ginger in large bowl; stir to blend. Remove half of mixture; cover and refrigerate. Add turkey to remaining mixture. Cover; marinate 2 hours in refrigerator, stirring occasionally.

2. Line large baking sheet with foil; spray with nonstick cooking spray. Remove turkey from marinade; discard marinade. Add remaining 1 tablespoon soy sauce to reserved half of marinade; whisk until smooth and well blended.

3. Set oven to broil. Alternately thread turkey, bell pepper and onion on four wooden or metal skewers. (If using wooden skewers, soak in water 20 to 30 minutes before using to prevent them from burning.) Place on prepared baking sheet.

4. Broil 4 inches from heat source 3 minutes. Brush evenly with reserved marinade mixture. Broil 6 to 9 minutes or until turkey is no longer pink.

5. Spoon ¼ cup brown rice onto four plates. Top each with 1 skewer.

---

nutritionals

Serving Size: *1 kabob and ¼ cup rice*, Calories: *190*, Total Fat: *2g*, Saturated Fat: *0g*, Cholesterol: *35mg*, Sodium: *510mg*, Carbohydrate: *20g*, Dietary Fiber: *2g*, Sugar: *7g*, Protein: *24g*

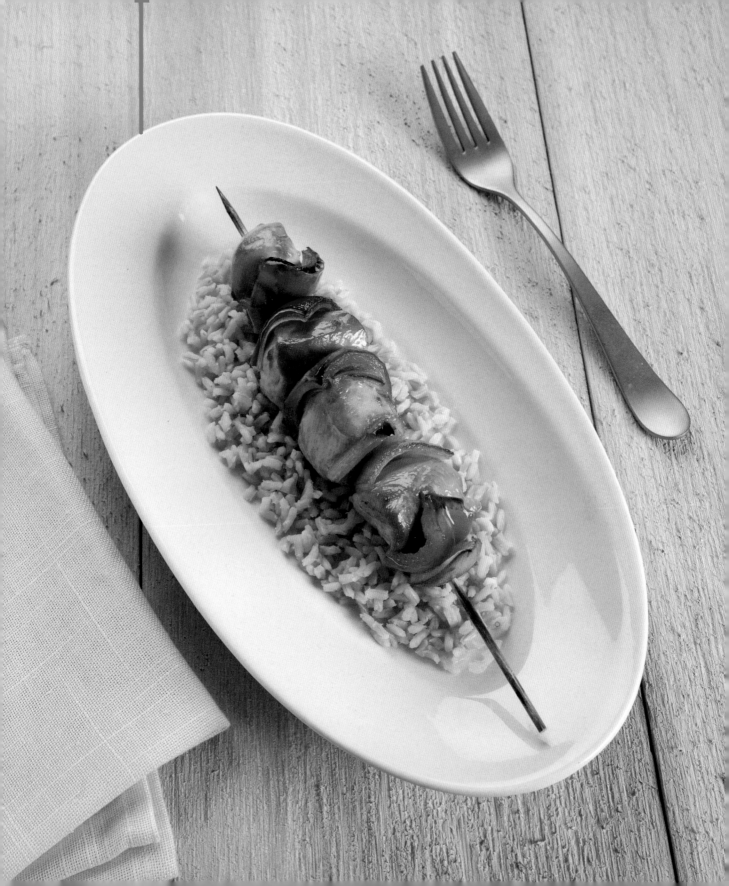

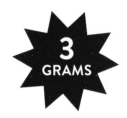

3 GRAMS

THAI DUCK WITH BEANS AND SPROUTS

makes 4 servings

Juice of 1 lime (about 2 tablespoons)

2 tablespoons vegetable oil, divided

2 tablespoons soy sauce

1 tablespoon fish sauce

2 teaspoons minced fresh ginger

2 cloves garlic, minced

1 pound boneless skinless duck breast, cut into ¼-inch strips

3 cups fresh green beans

1 cup chicken broth

4 green onions, cut into 1-inch pieces

1½ cups bean sprouts

1. Combine lime juice, 1 tablespoon oil, soy sauce, fish sauce, ginger and garlic in medium bowl; stir to blend. Add duck; toss to coat. Cover; refrigerate 30 minutes to 8 hours.

2. Heat remaining 1 tablespoon oil in wok or large skillet over high heat. Remove duck from marinade; reserve marinade. Add duck to wok; stir-fry 4 minutes or until no longer pink. Remove duck from wok with slotted spoon.

3. Add green beans to wok; stir-fry 5 to 6 minutes or until green beans are almost cooked. Add broth, green onions and reserved marinade to wok; boil 2 minutes. Return duck and accumulated juices to wok. Add bean sprouts; cook and stir until heated through.

nutritionals

Serving Size: *4 ounces*, Calories: *260*, Total Fat: *12g*, Saturated Fat: *3g*, Cholesterol: *85mg*, Sodium: *1130mg*, Carbohydrate: *11g*, Dietary Fiber: *2g*, Sugar: *3g*, Protein: *28g*

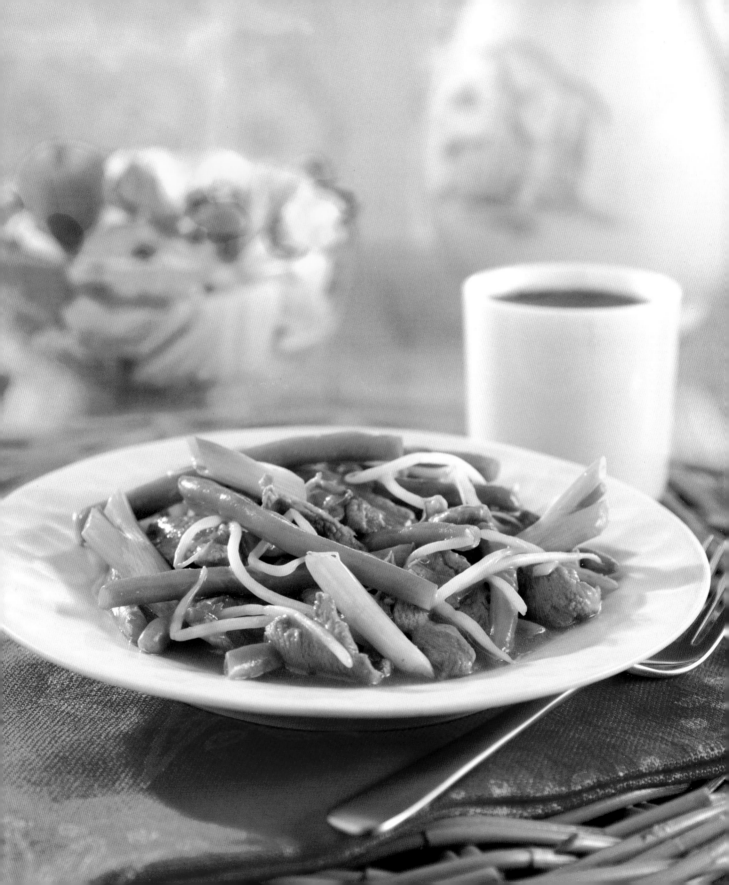

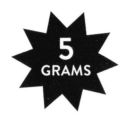

5 GRAMS

CANNELLINI CHICKEN SKILLET

makes 4 servings

2   tablespoons olive oil

2   boneless skinless chicken breasts, cut into 1-inch chunks

1   can (about 14 ounces) diced tomatoes

1   cup frozen chopped spinach

2   cloves garlic, chopped

1   tablespoon chopped fresh rosemary leaves or 1 teaspoon dried rosemary

1   teaspoon salt

½   teaspoon red pepper flakes

1   can (about 15 ounces) cannellini beans, rinsed and drained

1   cup grape tomatoes, cut in half

1. Heat oil in large skillet over medium-high heat. Add chicken; cook and stir 8 minutes or until chicken is cooked through.

2. Add diced tomatoes, spinach, garlic, rosemary, salt and red pepper flakes to skillet; cook and stir 10 minutes or until spinach is thawed. Add beans and grape tomatoes; cook 2 minutes or until beans are heated through.

nutritionals

Serving Size: *about 1½ cups*, Calories: *280*, Total Fat: *9g*, Saturated Fat: *2g*, Cholesterol: *45mg*, Sodium: *1240mg*, Carbohydrate: *28g*, Dietary Fiber: *9g*, Sugar: *5g*, Protein: *23g*

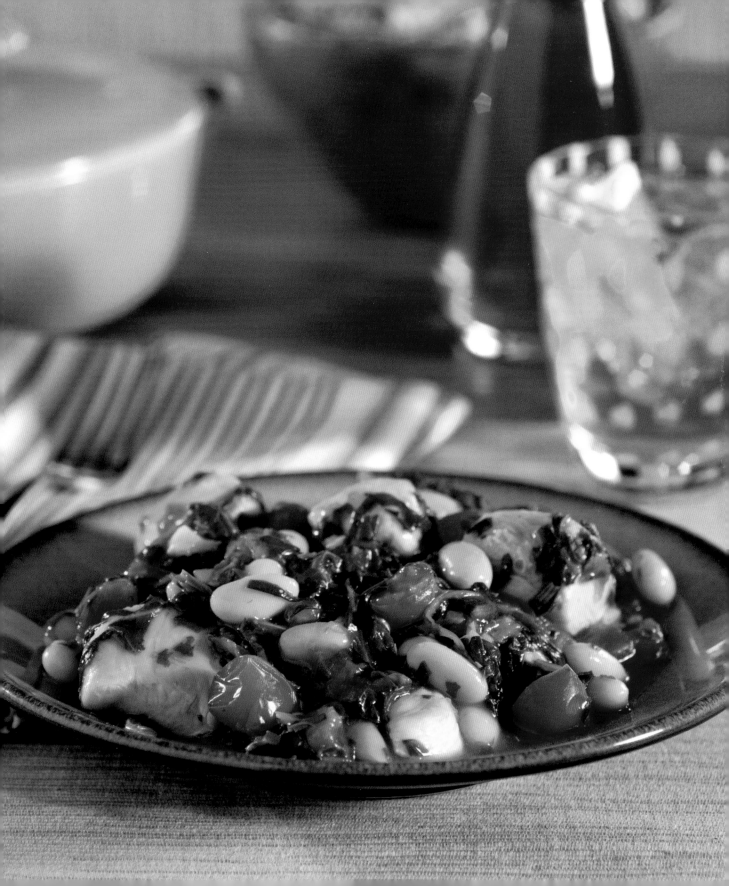

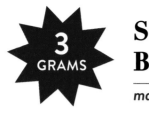

3 GRAMS

SOUTHWESTERN TURKEY BREAST

makes 6 servings

1   can (about 15 ounces) black beans, rinsed and drained

1   can (about 14 ounces) fire-roasted diced tomatoes

1   large onion, coarsely chopped

1   canned chipotle pepper in adobo sauce, chopped

1¼ teaspoons ground cumin, divided

1¼ teaspoons ground coriander, divided

¾   teaspoon ground cinnamon, divided

½   teaspoon salt

1   whole bone-in turkey breast (6 to 7 pounds), skin removed

¼   cup fresh cilantro, chopped

2   teaspoons fresh lime juice

1   teaspoon grated lime peel, finely chopped

Lime wedges (optional)

SLOW COOKER DIRECTIONS

1. Stir beans, tomatoes, onion, chipotle pepper, 1 teaspoon cumin, 1 teaspoon coriander, ½ teaspoon cinnamon and salt into slow cooker. Place turkey on top. Cover; cook on LOW 6 hours or on HIGH 3 hours or until turkey is cooked through (160°F).

2. Remove turkey. Stir remaining ¼ teaspoon cumin, ¼ teaspoon coriander, ¼ teaspoon cinnamon, cilantro, lime juice and lime peel into slow cooker. Serve bean mixture alongside turkey. Garnish with lime wedges.

nutritionals

Serving Size: *4 ounces turkey with about ¾ cup bean mixture*, Calories: *270*, Total Fat: *11g*, Saturated Fat: *3g*, Cholesterol: *70mg*, Sodium: *720mg*, Carbohydrate: *16g*, Dietary Fiber: *4g*, Sugar: *3g*, Protein: *26g*

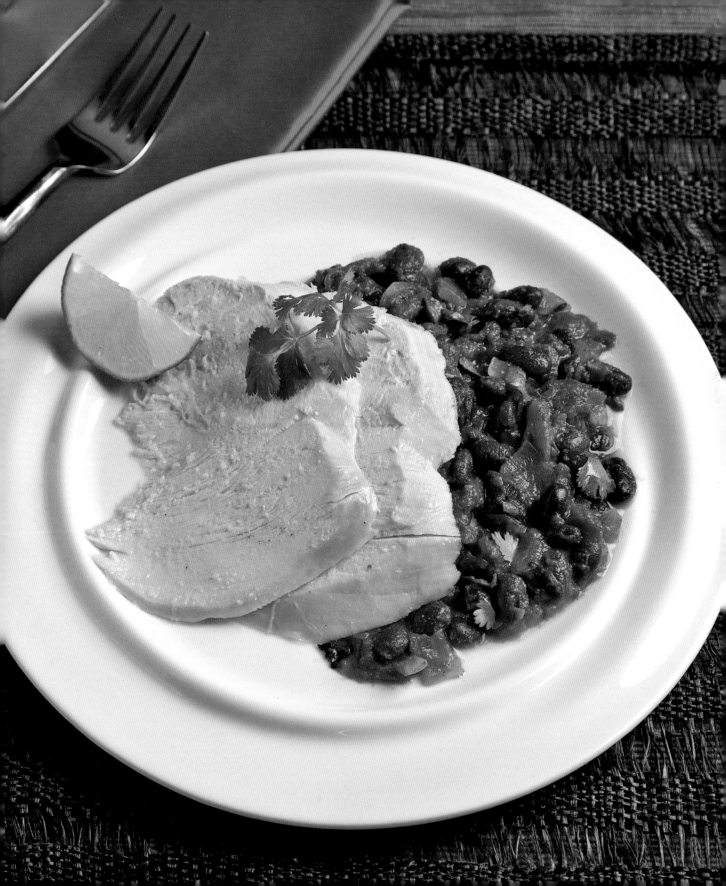

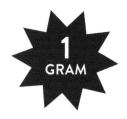

1 GRAM

SPICED CHICKEN SKEWERS WITH YOGURT-TAHINI SAUCE

makes 8 servings

1 cup plain nonfat Greek yogurt

¼ cup chopped fresh parsley, plus additional for garnish

¼ cup tahini

2 tablespoons lemon juice

1 clove garlic

¾ teaspoon salt, divided

1 tablespoon vegetable oil

2 teaspoons garam masala

1 pound boneless skinless chicken breasts, cut into 1-inch pieces

1. Spray grill grid with nonstick cooking spray. Prepare grill for direct cooking.

2. For yogurt-tahini sauce, combine yogurt, ¼ cup parsley, tahini, lemon juice, garlic and ¼ teaspoon salt in food processor or blender; process until combined. Set aside.

3. Combine oil, garam masala and remaining ½ teaspoon salt in medium bowl. Add chicken; toss to coat evenly. Thread chicken on eight 6-inch wooden or metal skewers. (If using wooden skewers, soak in water 20 to 30 minutes before using to prevent them from burning.)

4. Grill chicken skewers over medium-high heat 5 minutes per side or until chicken is no longer pink. Serve with yogurt-tahini sauce. Garnish with additional parsley.

nutritionals

Serving Size: *1 skewer with about 2 tablespoons sauce*, Calories: *145*, Total Fat: *7g*, Saturated Fat: *1g*, Cholesterol: *38mg*, Sodium: *285mg*, Carbohydrate: *4g*, Dietary Fiber: *0g*, Sugar: *1g*, Protein: *16g*

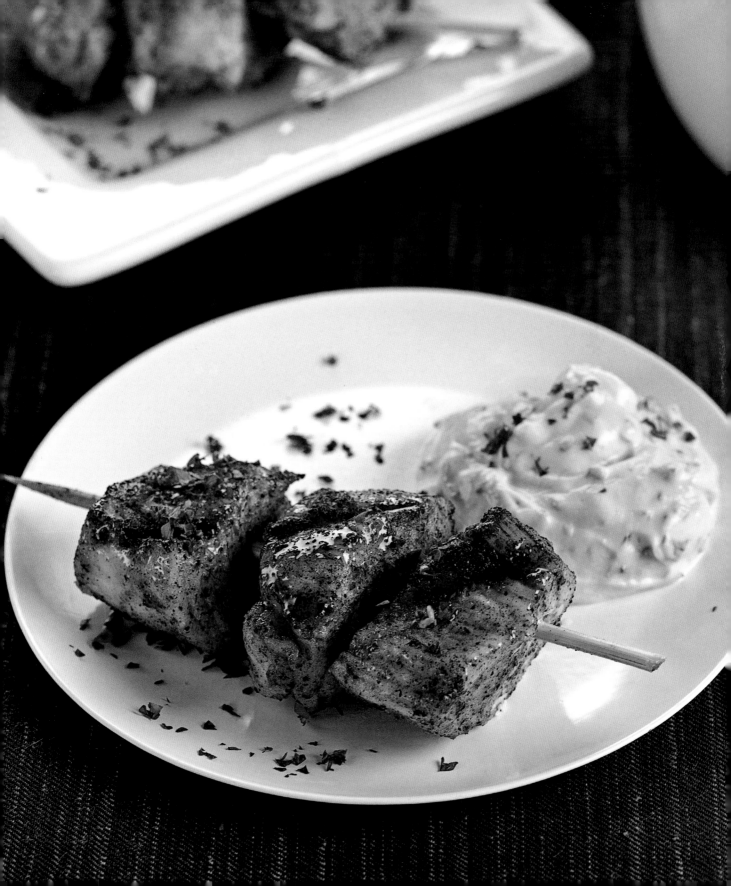

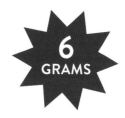

6 GRAMS

ASIAN LETTUCE WRAPS WITH HOISIN DIPPING SAUCE

makes 4 servings

2 tablespoons hoisin sauce

2 tablespoons pomegranate juice

½ teaspoon grated orange peel

2 cups coleslaw mix or broccoli slaw mix

¾ cup frozen shelled edamame, thawed

½ cup matchstick carrots

2 tablespoons chopped fresh cilantro

½ medium jalapeño pepper,* seeded and sliced into thin strips

1½ cups cooked diced chicken

1 ounce toasted peanuts

12 Bibb lettuce leaves or romaine leaves

Jalapeño peppers can sting and irritate the skin, so wear rubber gloves when handling peppers and do not touch your eyes.

1. Combine hoisin sauce, pomegranate juice and orange peel in small bowl; set aside.

2. Combine coleslaw, edamame, carrots, cilantro and jalapeño pepper in medium bowl. Add chicken and peanuts; toss gently.

3. Arrange lettuce leaves on large plate. Spoon about ⅓ cup chicken mixture on top of each lettuce leaf and drizzle with 1 teaspoon sauce.

nutritionals

Serving Size: *3 wraps*, Calories: *220*, Total Fat: *6g*, Saturated Fat: *2g*, Cholesterol: *45mg*, Sodium: *220mg*, Carbohydrate: *11g*, Dietary Fiber: *2g*, Sugar: *6g*, Protein: *30g*

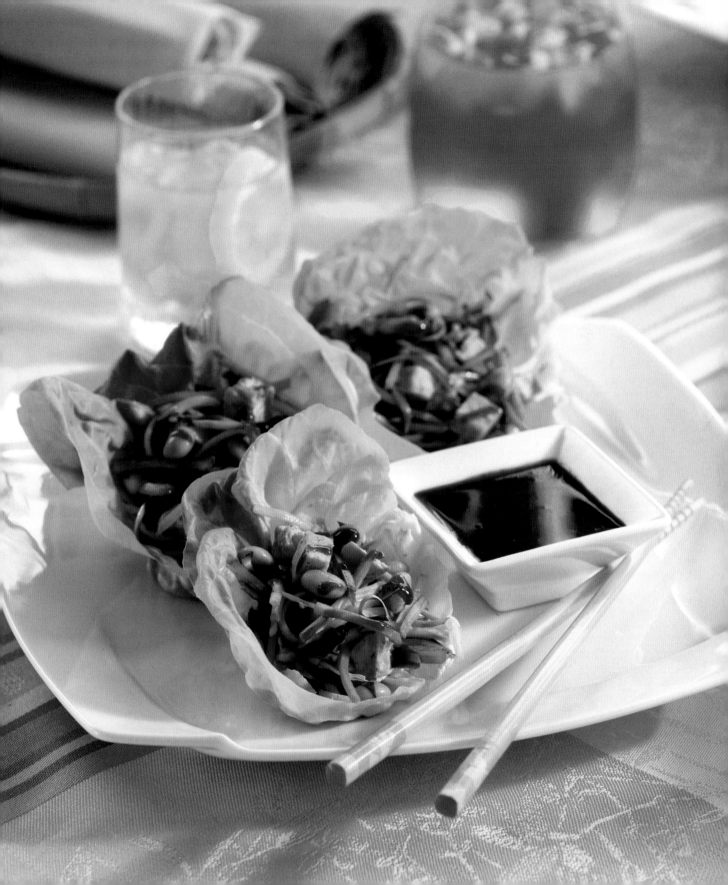

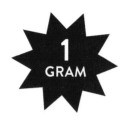

1 GRAM

CHICKEN PISTACHIO

makes 4 servings

4   boneless skinless chicken breasts

4   sheets (18×12 inches each) heavy duty foil, lightly sprayed with nonstick cooking spray

1   tablespoon olive oil

¼   teaspoon paprika

¼   cup finely chopped pistachio nuts

2   tablespoons finely chopped green onion

Lemon slices (optional)

1. Preheat oven to 375°F. Place chicken breasts on foil sheets. Brush chicken with oil; sprinkle with paprika. Double fold sides and ends of foil to seal packets, leaving head space for heat circulation. Place packets on baking sheet.

2. Bake packets 25 minutes. Remove from oven. Carefully open one end of foil packet to allow steam to escape. Open foil completely; sprinkle chicken with pistachios and green onion. Leave foil open and return to oven. Bake 5 minutes or until chicken is no longer pink in center (165°F).

3. Transfer contents of packets to serving plates. Garnish with lemon slices.

nutritionals

Serving Size: *1 packet*, Calories: *220*, Total Fat: *10g*, Saturated Fat: *2g*, Cholesterol: *85mg*, Sodium: *55mg*, Carbohydrate: *2g*, Dietary Fiber: *1g*, Sugar: *1g*, Protein: *28g*

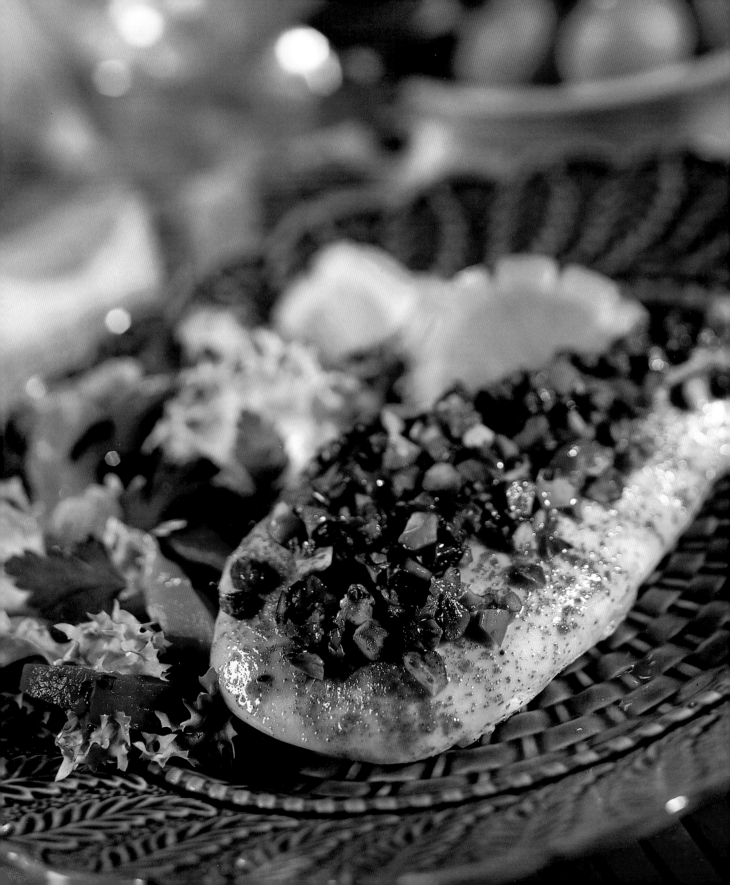

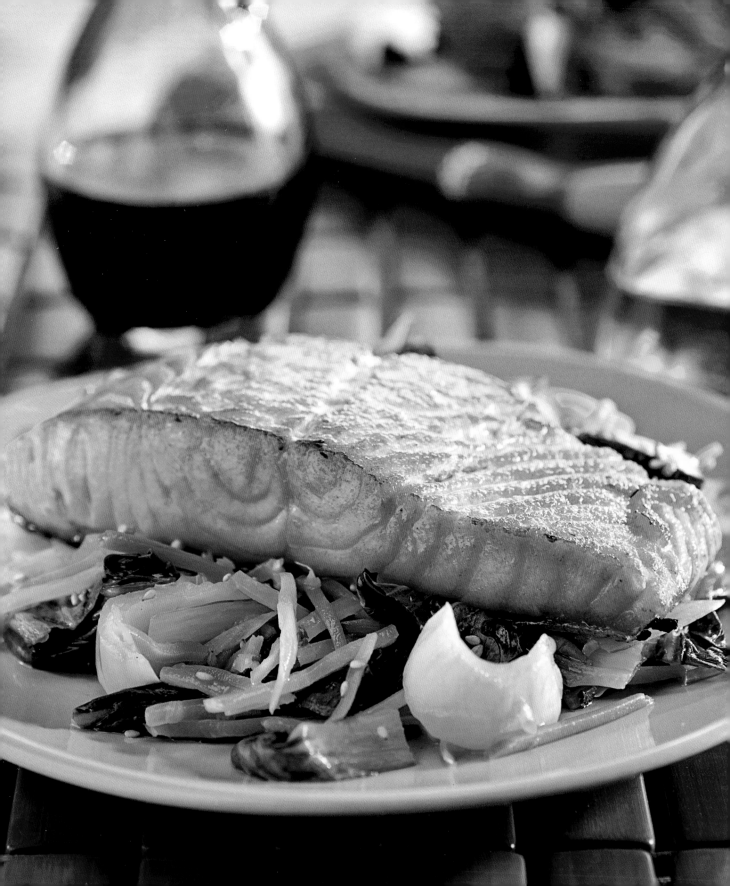

SEAFOOD

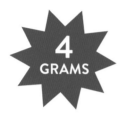

4 GRAMS

PAN-COOKED BOK CHOY SALMON

makes 2 servings

1 pound bok choy or napa cabbage, chopped

1 cup broccoli slaw mix

2 tablespoons olive oil, divided

2 salmon fillets (4 to 6 ounces each)

¼ teaspoon salt

½ teaspoon black pepper

1 teaspoon sesame seeds

1. Combine bok choy and broccoli slaw mix in colander; rinse and drain well.

2. Heat 1 tablespoon oil in large skillet over medium heat. Sprinkle salmon with salt and pepper. Add salmon to skillet; cook 3 minutes per side. Remove salmon from skillet.

3. Add remaining 1 tablespoon oil and sesame seeds to skillet; stir to toast sesame seeds. Add bok choy mixture; cook and stir 3 to 4 minutes.

4. Return salmon to skillet. Reduce heat to low; cover and cook 4 minutes or until salmon begins to flake when tested with fork. Season with additional salt and pepper, if desired.

nutritionals

Serving Size: *½ of recipe*, Calories: *410*, Total Fat: *30g*, Saturated Fat: *6g*, Cholesterol: *60mg*, Sodium: *520mg*, Carbohydrate: *8g*, Dietary Fiber: *3g*, Sugar: *4g*, Protein: *28g*

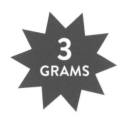

3 GRAMS

LEMON ROSEMARY SHRIMP AND VEGETABLE SOUVLAKI

makes 4 kabobs

8 ounces large raw shrimp, peeled and deveined (with tails on)

1 medium zucchini, halved lengthwise and cut into ½-inch slices

½ medium red bell pepper, cut into 1-inch squares

8 green onions, trimmed and cut into 2-inch pieces

2 tablespoons extra virgin olive oil

2 tablespoons lemon juice

2 teaspoons grated lemon peel

2 medium cloves garlic, minced

½ teaspoon salt

½ teaspoon fresh rosemary

⅛ teaspoon red pepper flakes

1. Prepare grill for direct cooking. Spray grid or grill pan with nonstick cooking spray.

2. Spray four 12-inch bamboo or metal skewers with cooking spray. (If using bamboo skewers, soak in water 20 to 30 minutes before using to prevent them from burning.) Alternately thread shrimp, zucchini, bell pepper and green onions onto skewers. Spray skewers lightly with cooking spray.

3. Combine oil, lemon juice, lemon peel, garlic, salt, rosemary and red pepper flakes in small bowl; mix well.

4. Grill skewers over high heat 2 minutes per side. Remove to large serving platter; drizzle with sauce.

NOTE: "Souvlaki" is the Greek word for shishkebab. Souvlaki traditionally consists of fish or meat that has been seasoned in a mixture of oil, lemon juice and seasonings. Many souvlaki recipes, including this one, also include chunks of vegetables such as bell pepper and onion.

---

nutritionals

Serving Size: *1 kabob with 1 tablespoon sauce*, Calories: *130*, Total Fat: *8g*, Saturated Fat: *1g*, Cholesterol: *70mg*, Sodium: *630mg*, Carbohydrate: *6g*, Dietary Fiber: *2g*, Sugar: *3g*, Protein: *9g*

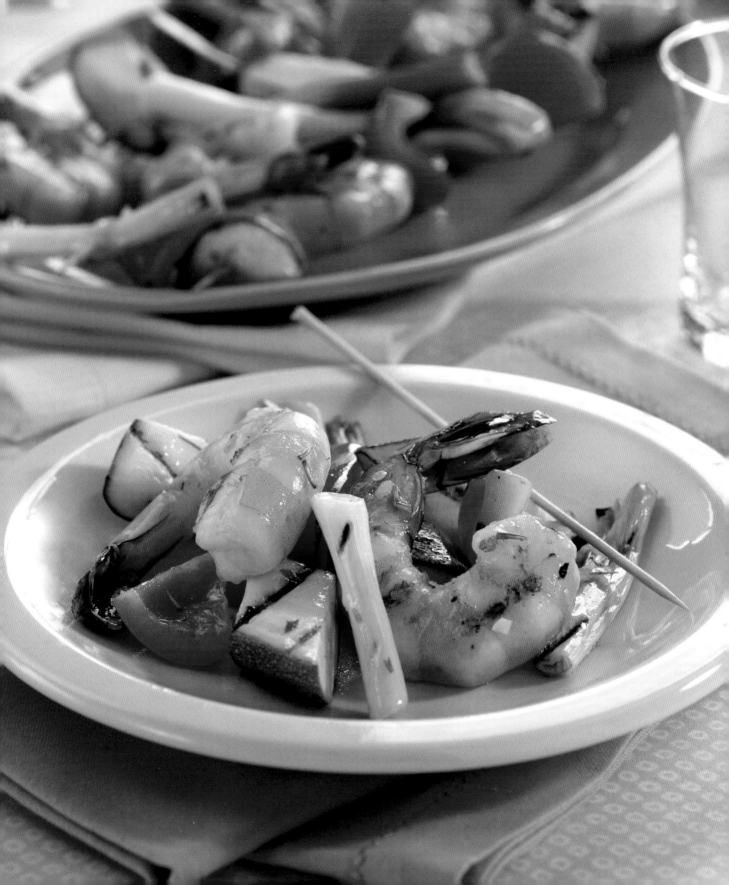

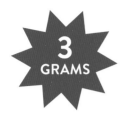

3 GRAMS

SALMON WITH BROWN RICE AND VEGETABLES

makes 4 servings

2 cups water

12 ounces skinless salmon fillets

2 cups sliced asparagus (1-inch pieces)

2 cups cooked brown rice

1 cup spinach, sliced into ½-inch strips

⅓ cup chicken broth

2 tablespoons chopped fresh chives

2 tablespoons fresh lemon juice

⅛ teaspoon black pepper

1. Bring water to a boil in large skillet over high heat. Add salmon; reduce heat to medium-low. Cover; simmer 10 minutes or until salmon begins to flake when tested with fork. Remove salmon from skillet; cut into large pieces when cool enough to handle.

2. Spray separate large skillet with nonstick cooking spray; heat over medium-high heat. Add asparagus; cook and stir 6 minutes or until tender. Stir in rice, spinach and broth. Reduce heat to low. Cover; cook 1 to 2 minutes or until spinach is wilted and rice is heated through. Stir in salmon, chives, lemon juice and pepper.

nutritionals

Serving Size: *about 1⅓ cups*, Calories: *320*, Total Fat: *12g*, Saturated Fat: *3g*, Cholesterol: *45mg*, Sodium: *140mg*, Carbohydrate: *29g*, Dietary Fiber: *5g*, Sugar: *3g*, Protein: *22g*

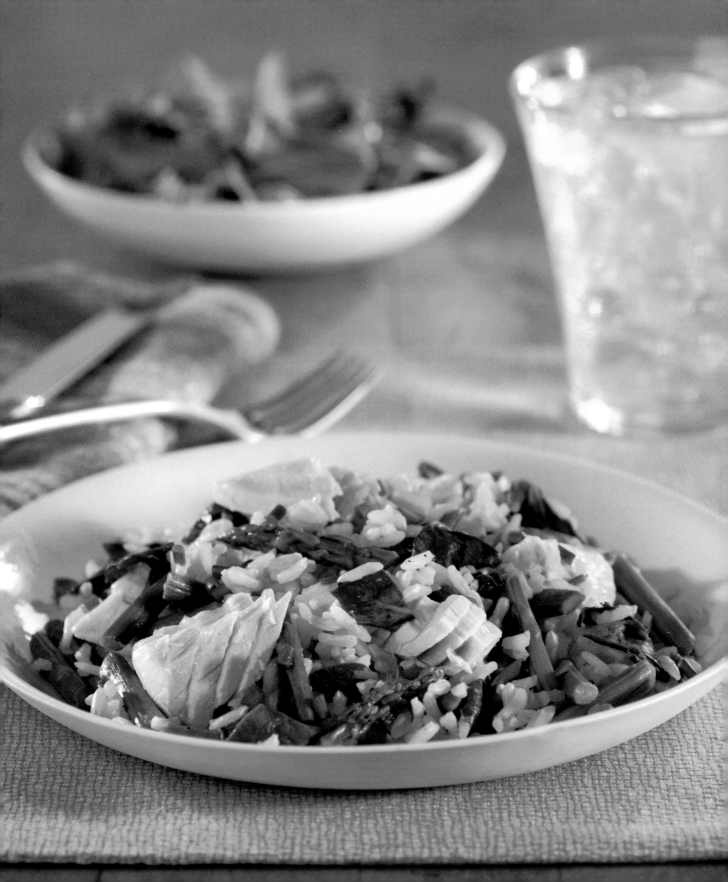

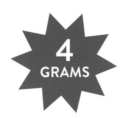

4 GRAMS

GRILLED TUNA WITH CHICKPEA SALAD

makes 4 servings

2 tablespoons fresh lime juice

3 teaspoons Dijon mustard, divided

3 teaspoons olive oil, divided

½ teaspoon black pepper, divided

2 tablespoons minced fresh chives, divided

2 tuna steaks (6 ounces each), 1 inch thick

1 large red bell pepper, diced

1 can (about 15 ounces) chickpeas, rinsed and drained

1 medium jalapeño pepper,* minced

1 large shallot, minced

2 tablespoons chicken broth

1 teaspoon lemon juice

¼ teaspoon salt

⅛ teaspoon dried oregano

Lemon or lime wedges (optional)

Jalapeño peppers can sting and irritate the skin, so wear rubber gloves when handling peppers and do not touch your eyes.

1. Combine lime juice, 1 teaspoon mustard, 1 teaspoon oil, ¼ teaspoon black pepper and 1 tablespoon chives in shallow bowl. Add tuna; turn to coat. Marinate at room temperature 30 minutes.

2. Meanwhile, combine bell pepper, chickpeas, jalapeño pepper and shallot in medium bowl. Stir together remaining 2 teaspoons oil, broth, lemon juice, remaining 2 teaspoons mustard, salt, remaining ¼ teaspoon black pepper and oregano in small bowl. Pour over bean mixture; stir well.

3. Coat large skillet with nonstick cooking spray; heat over medium-high heat. Cook tuna 5 minutes per side or until done, but slightly pink in center. (Tuna will continue to cook when removed from heat.)

4. Cut each tuna steak in half. Sprinkle with remaining 1 tablespoon chives. Garnish with lemon or lime wedges. Serve salad on top of 3 to 4 spinach leaves, if desired, and alongside tuna.

---

nutritionals

Serving Size: *3 ounces tuna and ½ cup salad,* Calories: *270,* Total Fat: *9g,* Saturated Fat: *2g,* Cholesterol: *30mg,* Sodium: *540mg,* Carbohydrate: *20g,* Dietary Fiber: *5g,* Sugar: *4g,* Protein: *25g*

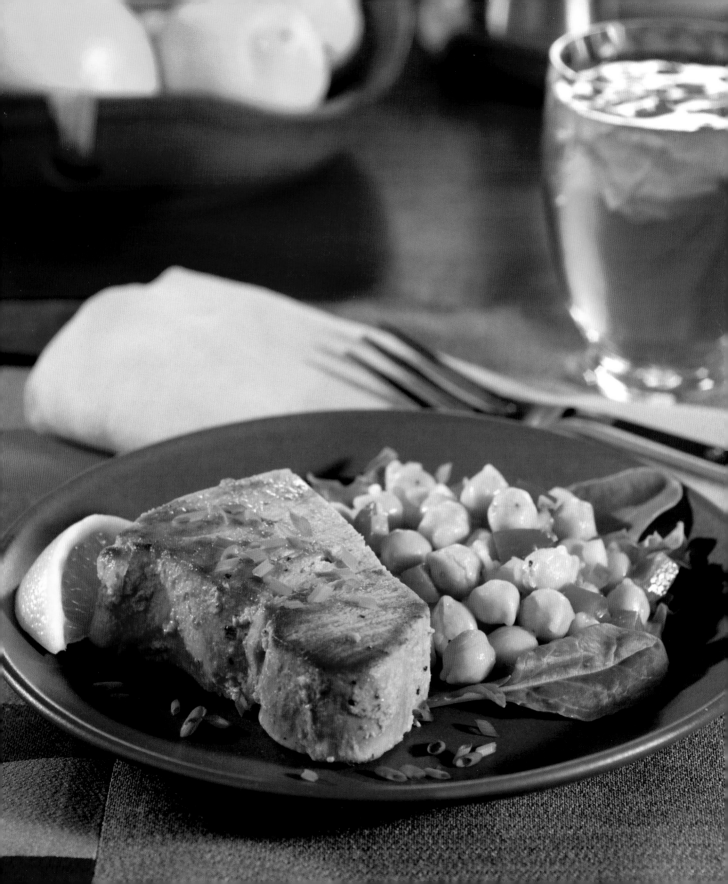

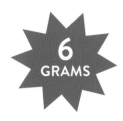

6 GRAMS

ROASTED SALMON WITH STRAWBERRY-ORANGE SALSA

makes 4 servings

4   salmon fillets (about ¼ pound each), skin removed

½   teaspoon ground cumin

½   teaspoon dried thyme

¼   teaspoon salt

¼   teaspoon black pepper

1   medium orange

1   cup diced fresh strawberries

¼   cup finely chopped poblano pepper* or green bell pepper

2   tablespoons finely chopped fresh cilantro

½   teaspoon grated fresh ginger

Poblano peppers can sting and irritate the skin, so wear rubber gloves when handling peppers and do not touch your eyes.

1. Preheat oven to 400°F.

2. Line baking sheet with foil; spray with nonstick cooking spray. Place salmon on prepared baking sheet; sprinkle with cumin, thyme, salt and black pepper. Bake 12 to 14 minutes or until salmon begins to flake when tested with fork.

3. Grate orange peel to measure ½ teaspoon; place in medium bowl. Peel and section orange; coarsely chop orange sections. Add orange sections, strawberries, poblano pepper, cilantro and ginger to bowl; mix well. Serve salmon with salsa.

nutritionals

Serving Size: *3 ounces salmon with ⅓ cup salsa*, Calories: *270*, Total Fat: *15g*, Saturated Fat: *4g*, Cholesterol: *60mg*, Sodium: *220mg*, Carbohydrate: *9g*, Dietary Fiber: *2g*, Sugar: *6g*, Protein: *24g*

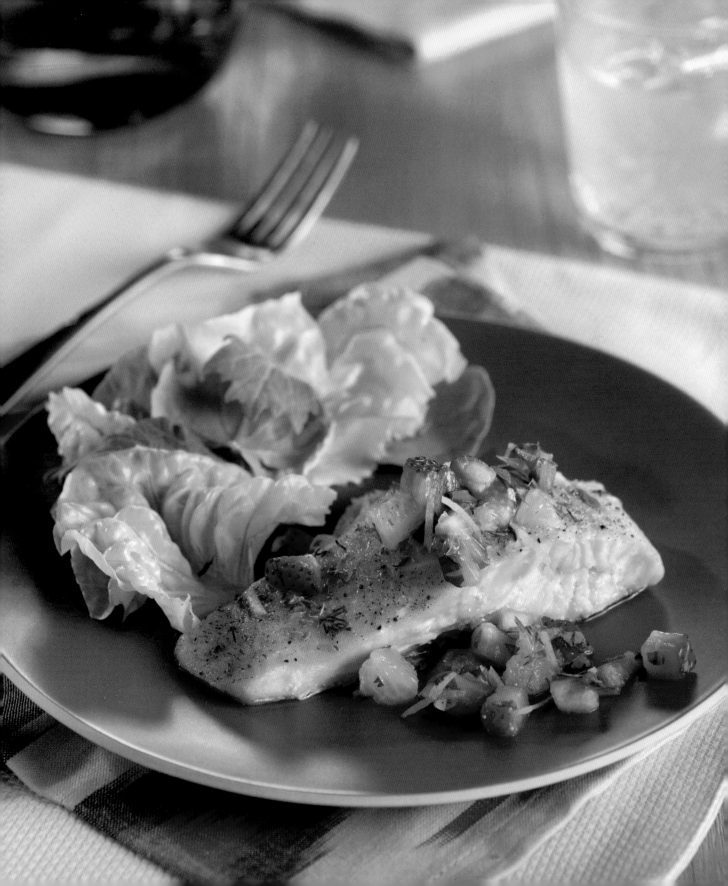

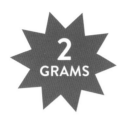
2 GRAMS

PESTO SCALLOP SKEWERS

makes 4 servings

1 to 2 red or yellow bell peppers, cut into bite-size pieces

16 jumbo sea scallops (about 1 pound)

2 tablespoons prepared pesto

1. Thread two bell pepper pieces and one scallop onto each of 16 short wooden or metal skewers. (If using wooden skewers, soak in water 20 to 30 minutes before using to prevent them from burning.) Brush pesto over bell peppers and scallops.

2. Heat nonstick grill pan or large nonstick skillet over medium-high heat. Cook skewers 2 to 3 minutes on each side or until scallops are opaque in center.

nutritionals

Serving Size: *4 skewers*, Calories: *120*, Total Fat: *4g*, Saturated Fat: *1g*, Cholesterol: *25mg*, Sodium: *540mg*, Carbohydrate: *7g*, Dietary Fiber: *1g*, Sugar: *2g*, Protein: *14g*

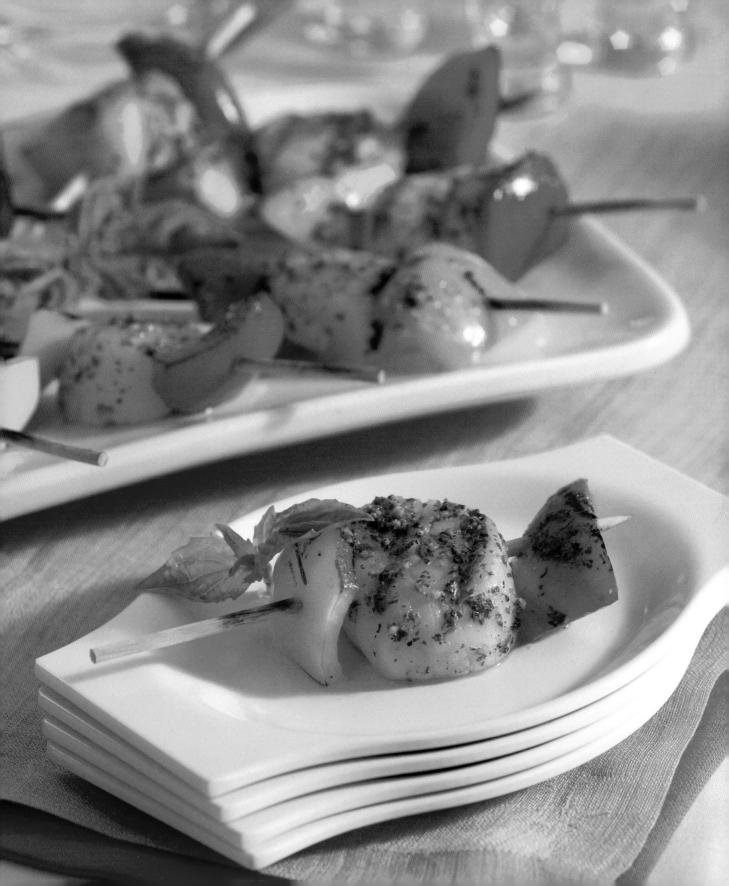

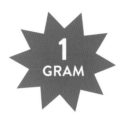

1 GRAM

DILLED SALMON IN PARCHMENT

makes 2 servings

2   skinless salmon fillets (4 to 6 ounces each)

2   tablespoons butter, melted

1   tablespoon lemon juice

1   tablespoon chopped fresh dill

1   tablespoon chopped shallots

Salt and black pepper

1. Preheat oven to 400°F. Cut two pieces of parchment paper into 12-inch squares; fold squares in half diagonally and cut into half heart shapes. Open parchment; place fish fillet on one side of each heart.

2. Combine butter and lemon juice in small bowl; drizzle over fish. Sprinkle with dill, shallots, salt and pepper to taste.

3. Fold parchment hearts in half. Beginning at top of heart, fold edges together, 2 inches at a time. At tip of heart, fold parchment over to seal.

4. Bake fish 10 minutes or until parchment pouch puffs up. To serve, cut an "X" through top layer of parchment and fold back points to display contents.

nutritionals

Serving Size: *½ of recipe*, Calories: *315*, Total Fat: *24g*, Saturated Fat: *10g*, Cholesterol: *88mg*, Sodium: *141mg*, Carbohydrate: *2g*, Dietary Fiber: *1g*, Sugar: *1g*, Protein: *23g*

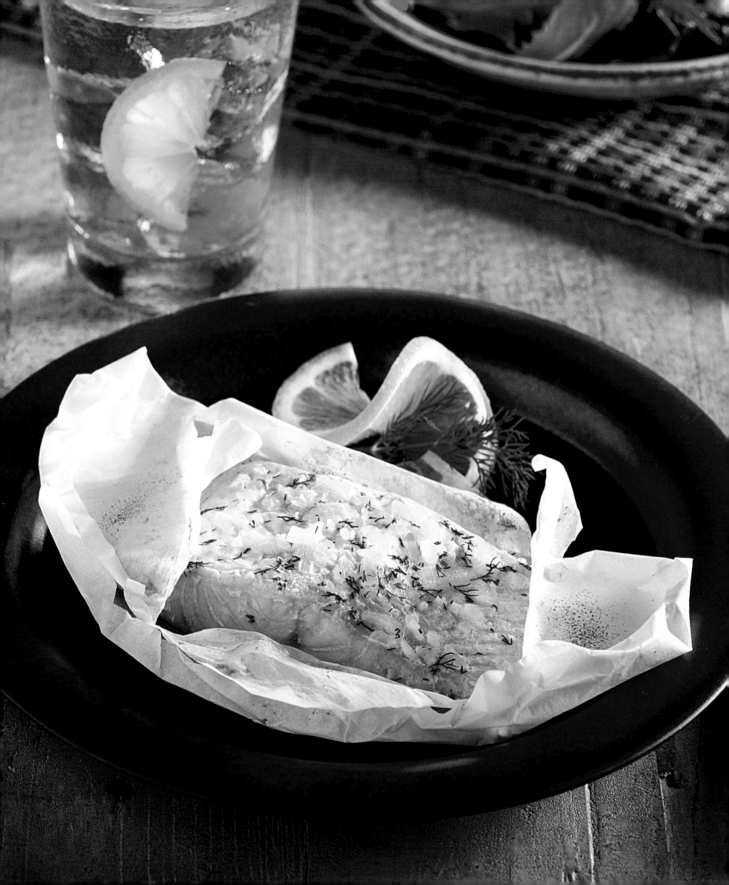

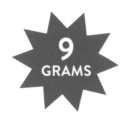
9 GRAMS

TUNA STEAKS WITH PINEAPPLE AND TOMATO SALSA

makes 4 servings

1 medium tomato, chopped

1 can (8 ounces) pineapple chunks in juice, drained and chopped

2 tablespoons chopped fresh cilantro

1 jalapeño pepper*, seeded and minced

1 tablespoon minced red onion

½ teaspoon grated lime peel

2 teaspoons lime juice

4 tuna steaks (4 ounces each)

½ teaspoon salt

⅛ teaspoon black pepper

2 teaspoons olive oil

*Jalapeño peppers can sting and irritate the skin, so wear rubber gloves when handling peppers and do not touch your eyes.

1. For salsa, combine tomato, pineapple, cilantro, jalapeño pepper, onion, lime peel and lime juice in medium bowl; stir to blend.

2. Sprinkle tuna with salt and black pepper. Heat oil in large nonstick skillet over medium-high heat. Add tuna; cook 2 to 3 minutes per side for medium rare or to desired degree of doneness. Serve with salsa.

---

nutritionals

Serving Size: *1 tuna steak with about ½ cup salsa,* Calories: *230,* Total Fat: *8g,* Saturated Fat: *2g,* Cholesterol: *45mg,* Sodium: *340mg,* Carbohydrate: *11g,* Dietary Fiber: *1g,* Sugar: *9g,* Protein: *27g*

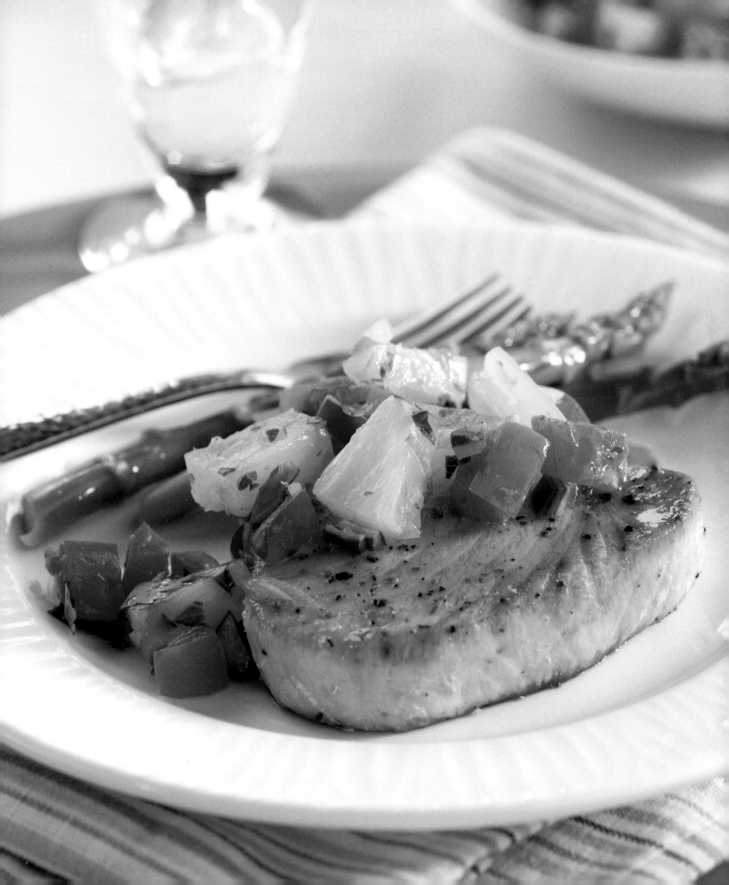

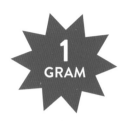

**1
GRAM**

HAZELNUT-COATED SALMON STEAKS

makes 4 servings

¼ cup hazelnuts

4 salmon steaks (about
    5 ounces each)

1 tablespoon apple butter

1 tablespoon Dijon mustard

¼ teaspoon dried thyme

⅛ teaspoon black pepper

1. Preheat oven to 375°F. Spread hazelnuts on ungreased baking sheet; bake 8 minutes or until lightly browned. Immediately transfer nuts to clean, dry dish towel. Fold towel over nuts; rub vigorously to remove as much of skins as possible. Finely chop hazelnuts in food processor or with knife.

2. *Increase oven temperature to 450°F.* Place salmon in single layer in baking dish. Combine apple butter, mustard, thyme and pepper in small bowl; brush over salmon. Top with hazelnuts, pressing to adhere.

3. Bake 14 to 16 minutes or until salmon begins to flake when tested with fork.

nutritionals

Serving Size: *1 salmon steak*, Calories: *350*, Total Fat: *23g*, Saturated Fat: *5g*, Cholesterol: *80mg*, Sodium: *170mg*, Carbohydrate: *2g*, Dietary Fiber: *1g*, Sugar: *1g*, Protein: *30g*

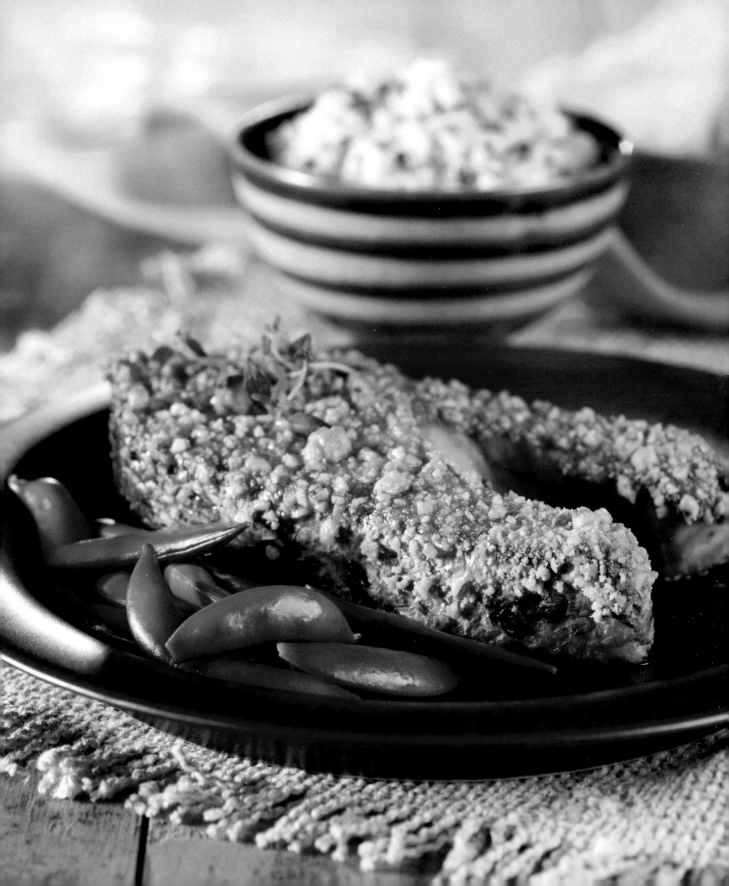

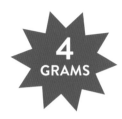

4 GRAMS

CALIFORNIA ROLL FARRO SUSHI BOWL

makes 6 servings

BOWL

1 package (8½ ounces) quick-cooking farro

2 tablespoons rice vinegar

½ teaspoon salt

1 cup shredded carrots

2 avocados, sliced

2 mini (kirby) cucumbers, thinly sliced

¾ pound crab sticks or imitation crab sticks

2 teaspoons toasted sesame seeds

DRESSING

⅓ cup mayonnaise

1 teaspoon sriracha sauce

1 teaspoon dark sesame oil

1 teaspoon rice vinegar

1. Prepare farro according to package directions.

2. Combine 2 tablespoons rice vinegar and salt in large microwavable bowl; microwave on HIGH 30 to 45 seconds or until salt is dissolved. Stir mixture; add farro and toss to coat.

3. Divide farro mixture evenly among six bowls. Top each with equal amount of carrots, avocados, cucumbers and crab sticks. Sprinkle with sesame seeds.

4. Whisk mayonnaise, sriracha sauce, sesame oil and 1 teaspoon rice vinegar in small bowl until well blended. Serve with farro bowls as dressing.

nutritionals

Serving Size: *1 cup with 1 tablespoon dressing*, Calories: *390*, Total Fat: *20g*, Saturated Fat: *3g*, Cholesterol: *55mg*, Sodium: *640mg*, Carbohydrate: *38g*, Dietary Fiber: *8g*, Sugar: *4g*, Protein: *18g*

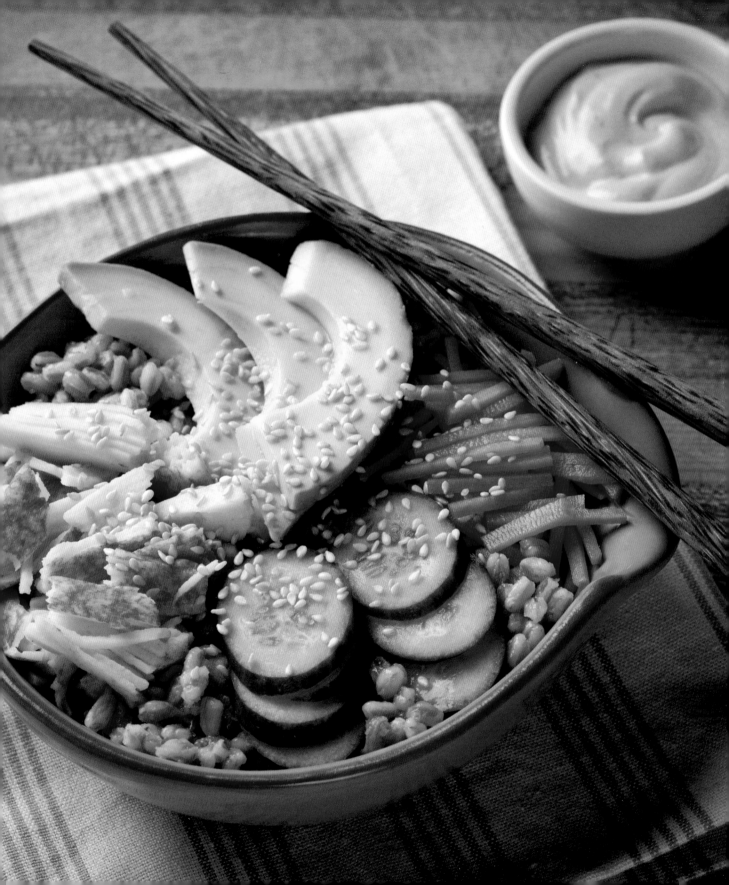

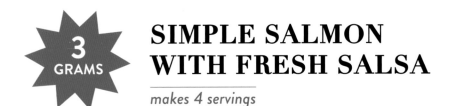

SIMPLE SALMON WITH FRESH SALSA

makes 4 servings

3 GRAMS

4   salmon fillets (about 4 ounces each), rinsed and patted dry

1   teaspoon salt, divided

½   teaspoon dried thyme

¼   teaspoon black pepper

½   cup chicken broth

1   medium cucumber, peeled, seeded and chopped

½   large green bell pepper, chopped

½   cup finely chopped radishes

½   cup quartered grape tomatoes

¼   cup chopped fresh cilantro

3   tablespoons fresh lime juice

2   tablespoons finely chopped red onion

    Hot cooked green beans (optional)

SLOW COOKER DIRECTIONS

1. Season salmon with ½ teaspoon salt, thyme and black pepper. Pour broth into slow cooker; add salmon. Cover; cook on LOW 3 hours.

2. Meanwhile, combine cucumber, bell pepper, radishes, tomatoes, cilantro, lime juice, onion and remaining ½ teaspoon salt in medium bowl. Cover; refrigerate until ready to serve.

3. To serve, place salmon on serving plates; top with salsa. Serve with green beans, if desired.

nutritionals

Serving Size: *1 salmon fillet with about ¾ cup salsa,* Calories: *260,* Total Fat: *15g,* Saturated Fat: *4g,* Cholesterol: *60mg,* Sodium: *790mg,* Carbohydrate: *7g,* Dietary Fiber: *2g,* Sugar: *3g,* Protein: *25g*

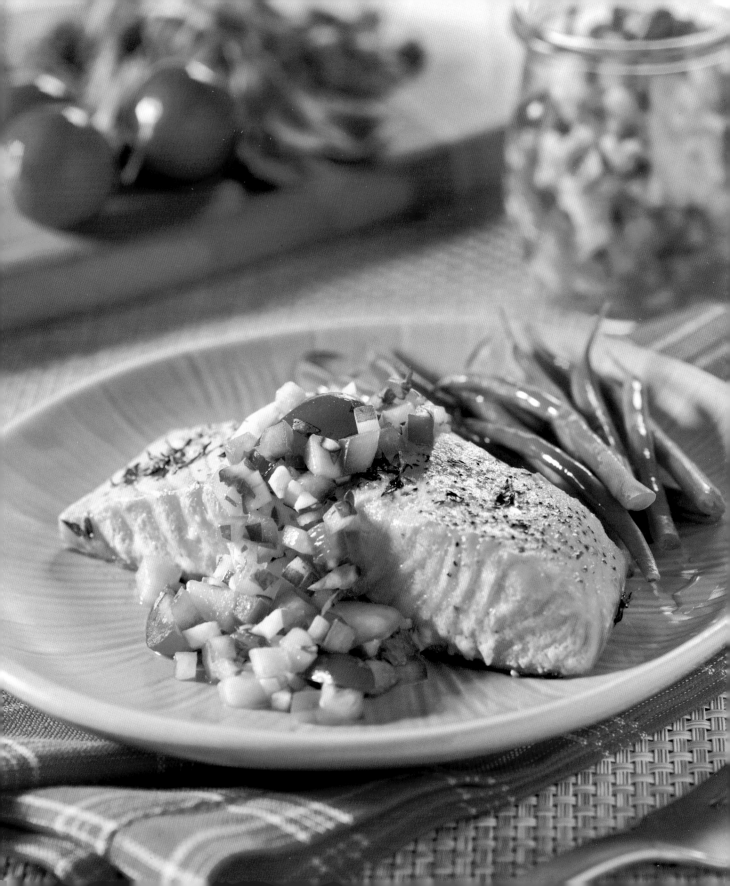

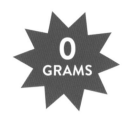

0 GRAMS

BOILED WHOLE LOBSTER WITH BUTTER SAUCE

makes 4 servings

½ cup (1 stick) butter

2 tablespoons chopped fresh parsley

1 tablespoon capers

1 tablespoon cider vinegar

2 live lobsters (1 pound total)

1. Fill 8-quart stockpot with enough water to cover lobsters. Cover stockpot; bring water to a boil over high heat. Melt butter in medium saucepan over medium heat. Cook and stir until butter turns dark chocolate brown. Remove from heat. Add parsley, capers and vinegar. Pour into two individual ramekins; set aside.

2. Holding each lobster by its back, submerge head first into boiling water. Cover and continue to heat. When water returns to a boil, cook lobsters 10 minutes.

3. Transfer to two large serving platters. Remove bands restraining claws. Cut through underside of shells with kitchen shears and loosen meat from shells. Provide nutcrackers and seafood forks. Serve lobsters with butter sauce.

NOTE: Purchase live lobsters as close to time of cooking as possible. Store in refrigerator until ready to cook.

---

nutritionals

Serving Size: *4 ounces lobster and 2 tablespoons butter sauce*, Calories: *310*, Total Fat: *24g*, Saturated Fat: *15g*, Cholesterol: *140mg*, Sodium: *670mg*, Carbohydrate: *2g*, Dietary Fiber: *0g*, Sugar: *0g*, Protein: *23g*

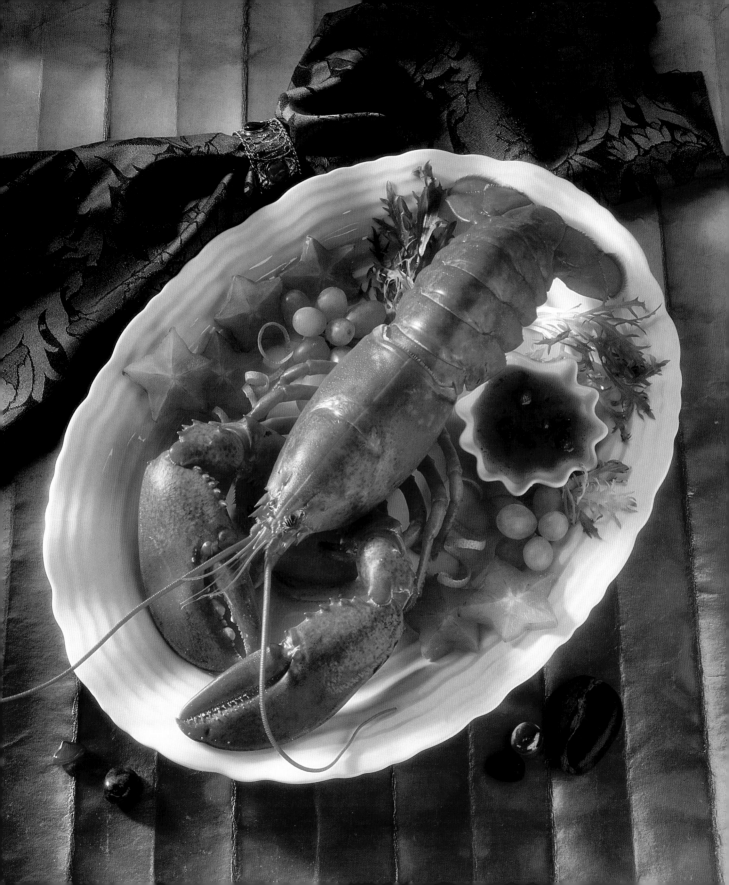

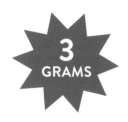

3 GRAMS

ROASTED SALMON AND ASPARAGUS WITH QUINOA

makes 4 servings

1 pound fresh thin asparagus spears

2½ teaspoons olive oil, divided

8 ounces wild-caught salmon fillet

1 teaspoon salt, divided

¼ teaspoon black pepper, divided

½ cup uncooked quinoa

1 cup water

1 green onion, chopped

1 teaspoon lemon juice

½ teaspoon minced fresh dill

4 lemon wedges (optional)

1. Preheat oven to 400°F. Place asparagus in large nonstick roasting pan. Drizzle with 1 teaspoon oil. Roast 10 minutes. Turn asparagus and push to one side of pan. Arrange salmon, skin side down, on other side. Brush with ½ teaspoon oil, sprinkle with ½ teaspoon salt and ⅛ teaspoon pepper. Roast 10 to 13 minutes or until salmon is cooked through. Remove asparagus and cut into bite-size pieces.

2. Meanwhile, place quinoa in fine-mesh strainer; rinse well under cold running water. Bring 1 cup water to a boil in small saucepan; stir in quinoa. Reduce heat to low; cover and simmer 10 to 15 minutes or until quinoa is tender and water is absorbed. Transfer to large bowl.

3. Stir in asparagus, green onion, remaining 1 teaspoon oil, ½ teaspoon salt, ⅛ teaspoon pepper, lemon juice and dill. Transfer to four plates; top with salmon. Garnish with lemon wedges.

nutritionals

Serving Size: *2 ounces salmon with ½ cup quinoa,* Calories: *220,* Total Fat: *8g,* Saturated Fat: *1g,* Cholesterol: *35mg,* Sodium: *620mg,* Carbohydrate: *19g,* Dietary Fiber: *4g,* Sugar: *3g,* Protein: *18g*

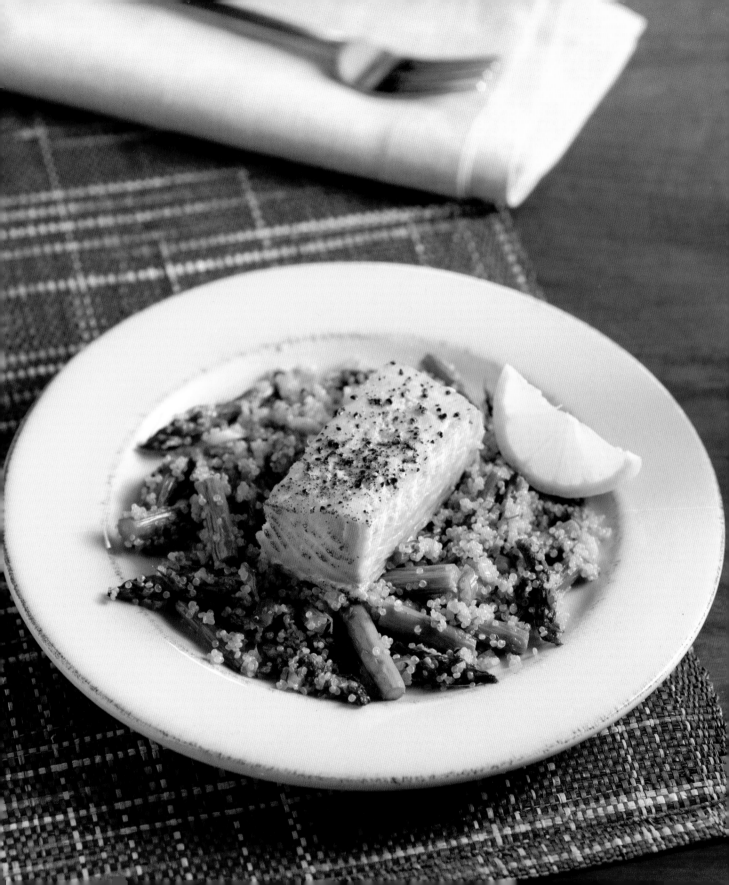

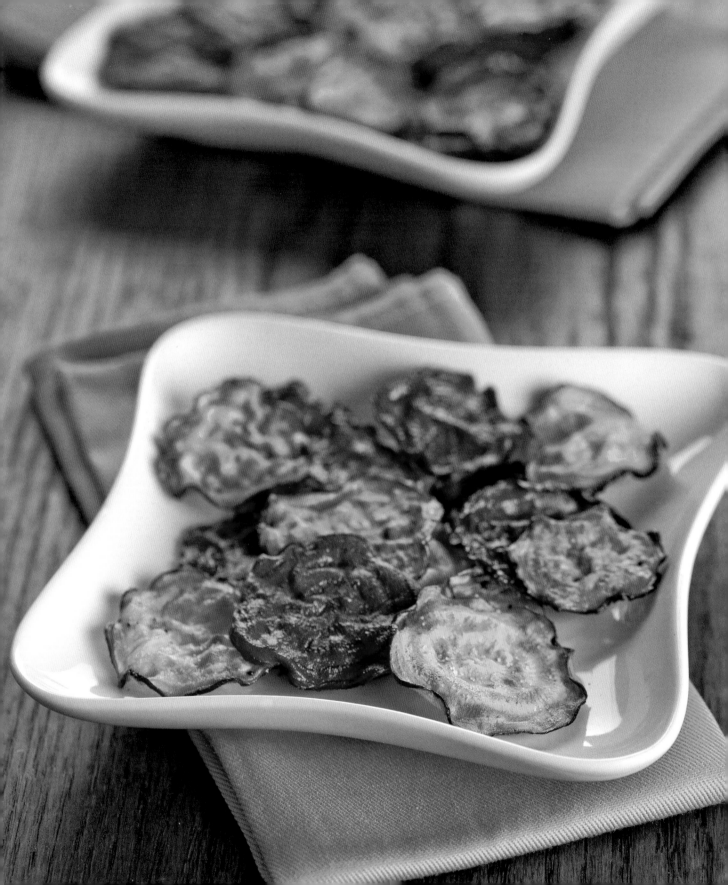

SNACKS

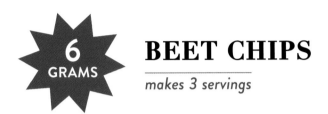

6 GRAMS

BEET CHIPS

makes 3 servings

3   medium beets (red and/or golden), trimmed

1½   tablespoons extra virgin olive oil

¼   teaspoon salt

¼   teaspoon black pepper

1. Preheat oven to 300°F.

2. Cut beets into very thin slices, about ⅟₁₆ inch thick. Combine beets, oil, salt and pepper in medium bowl; gently toss to coat. Arrange in single layer on baking sheets.

3. Bake 30 to 35 minutes or until darkened and crisp.* Spread on paper towels to cool completely.

*If the beet chips are darkened but not crisp, turn oven off and let chips stand in oven until crisp, about 10 minutes. Do not keep the oven on as the chips will burn easily.

nutritionals

Serving Size: *⅓ of recipe*, Calories: *100*, Total Fat: *7g*, Saturated Fat: *1g*, Cholesterol: *0mg*, Sodium: *260mg*, Carbohydrate: *8g*, Dietary Fiber: *2g*, Sugar: *6g*, Protein: *1g*

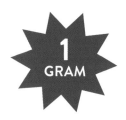

1 GRAM

COUNTRY FRENCH EGGS

makes 6 servings

6   hard-cooked eggs,
     peeled and sliced in half
     lengthwise

2   tablespoons milk

1   clove garlic, minced

1   tablespoon minced fresh
     tarragon *or* 1 teaspoon
     dried tarragon

⅛   teaspoon salt

⅛   teaspoon black pepper

2   teaspoons Dijon mustard

2   teaspoons tarragon vinegar

     Dash salt

     Dash black pepper

1   tablespoon olive oil

1   tablespoon butter

     Sprigs fresh tarragon
     (optional)

1. Remove yolks from egg halves. Mash yolks in small bowl. Add milk, garlic, minced tarragon, ⅛ teaspoon salt and ⅛ teaspoon pepper; mix well. Reserve 2 tablespoons yolk mixture. Fill egg halves with remaining yolk mixture, patting firmly into each egg.

2. For dressing, add mustard, vinegar, dash salt and dash pepper to reserved yolk mixture. Whisk in oil, pouring in thin stream; set aside.

3. Heat butter in large skillet over medium-low heat. Place egg halves, yolk-side down, in skillet. Cook 2 to 3 minutes or until yolk mixture is slightly golden. *Do not overcook.*

4. Pour dressing onto serving plate. Place cooked egg halves on plate over dressing. Garnish with tarragon sprigs.

---

nutritionals

Serving Size: *2 halves*, Calories: *120*, Total Fat: *10g*, Saturated Fat: *3g*, Cholesterol: *190mg*, Sodium: *220mg*, Carbohydrate: *1g*, Dietary Fiber: *0g*, Sugar: *1g*, Protein: *7g*

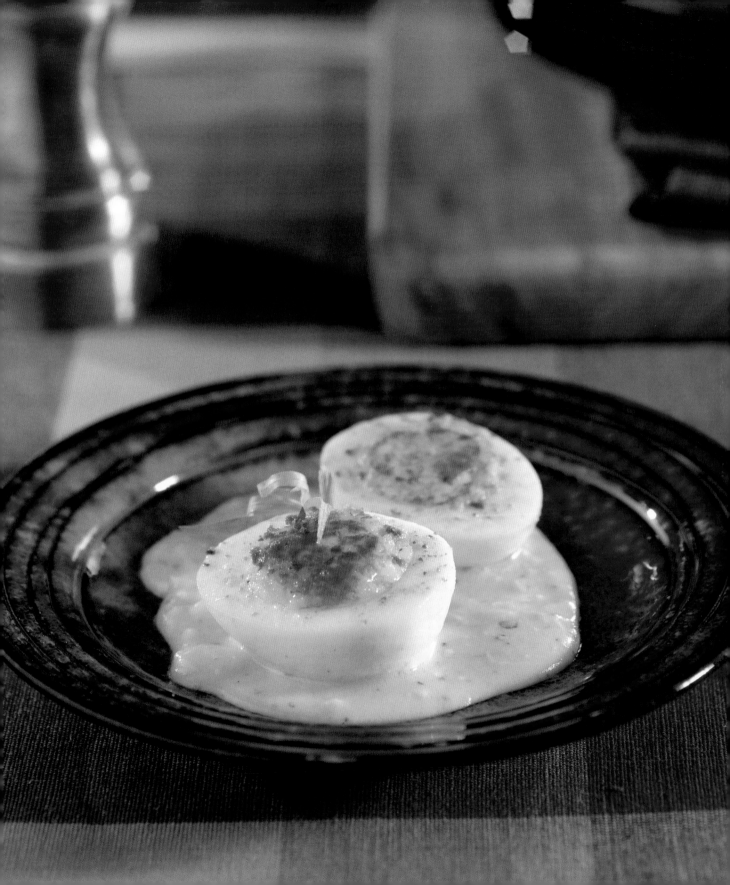

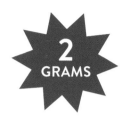

2 GRAMS

BARLEY "CAVIAR"

makes 4 servings

4   cups water

½   teaspoon salt, divided

¾   cup uncooked pearl barley

½   cup sliced pimiento-stuffed olives

½   cup finely chopped red bell pepper

1   stalk celery, chopped

1   large shallot, finely chopped

1   jalapeño pepper,* minced, or ¼ teaspoon red pepper flakes

2   tablespoons plus 1 teaspoon olive oil

4   teaspoons white wine vinegar

¼   teaspoon ground cumin

⅛   teaspoon black pepper

8   leaves endive or Bibb lettuce

Jalapeño peppers can sting and irritate the skin, so wear rubber gloves when handling peppers and do not touch your eyes.

1. Bring water and ¼ teaspoon salt to a boil in medium saucepan over high heat. Stir in barley. Reduce heat to low. Cover; simmer 45 minutes or until barley is tender. Remove from heat. Let stand 5 minutes. Rinse under cold running water; drain well. Place in large bowl.

2. Stir in olives, bell pepper, celery, shallot and jalapeño pepper. Stir together oil, vinegar, remaining ¼ teaspoon salt, cumin and black pepper in small bowl. Pour over barley mixture; stir gently to mix well. Let stand 10 minutes. To serve, spoon barley mixture evenly into endive leaves.

---

nutritionals

Serving Size: *2 filled endive leaves*, Calories: *250*, Total Fat: *11g*, Saturated Fat: *2g*, Cholesterol: *0mg*, Sodium: *800mg*, Carbohydrate: *35g*, Dietary Fiber: *7g*, Sugar: *2g*, Protein: *4g*

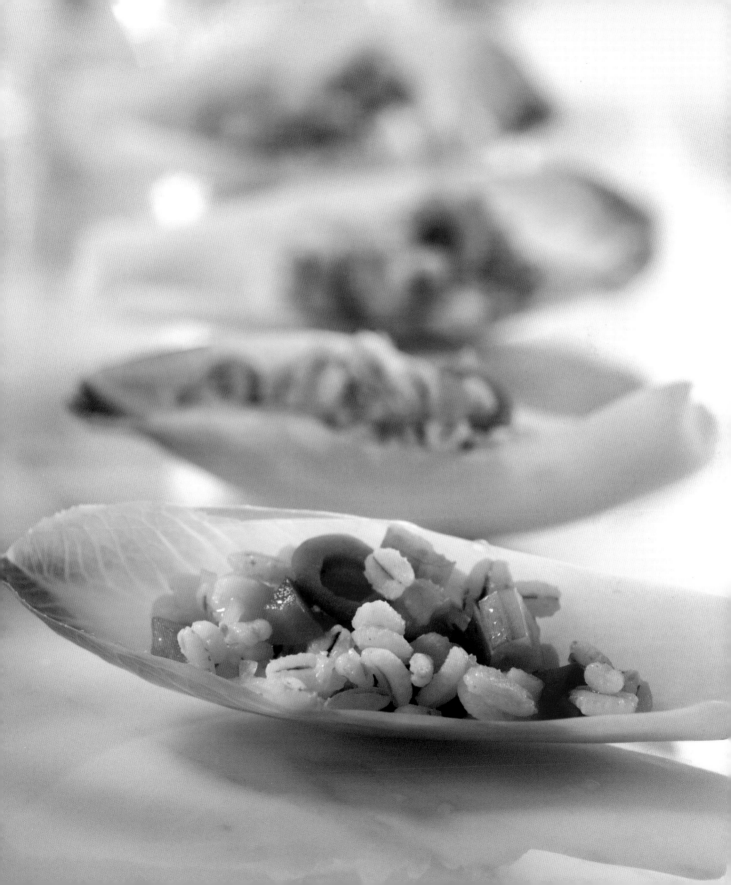

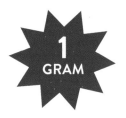

1 GRAM

CALIFORNIA HAM ROLLS

makes 4 servings

2 cups water

½ teaspoon salt, divided

1 cup uncooked short grain brown rice

2 tablespoons unseasoned rice vinegar* or cider vinegar

4 (8-inch) sheets sushi nori*

8 thin strips ham (about 4 ounces)

¼ cup soy sauce

1 tablespoon mirin (sweet rice wine)*

1 tablespoon minced fresh chives

These ingredients can be found in the Asian section of your supermarket.

1. Bring water and ¼ teaspoon salt to a boil in medium saucepan over high heat. Stir in rice. Reduce heat to low. Cover; simmer 40 to 45 minutes or until water is absorbed and rice is tender but chewy. Spoon rice into large shallow bowl.

2. Combine vinegar and remaining ¼ teaspoon salt in small bowl. Microwave on HIGH 30 seconds. Stir to dissolve salt. Pour over rice; stir to mix well. Set aside to cool.

3. Place 1 sheet of nori on work surface. Loosely spread about ½ cup rice over nori, leaving ½-inch border. Place 2 strips of ham along width of nori. Moisten top edge of nori sheet. Roll up tightly. Gently press to redistribute rice, if necessary. Cut into six slices with sharp knife. Place cut side up on serving plate. Repeat with remaining nori, rice and ham.

4. Combine soy sauce and mirin in small bowl. Sprinkle with chives. Serve with ham rolls.

nutritionals

Serving Size: *2 rolls*, Calories: *170*, Total Fat: *3g*, Saturated Fat: *0g*, Cholesterol: *15mg*, Sodium: *1200mg*, Carbohydrate: *28g*, Dietary Fiber: *3g*, Sugar: *1g*, Protein: *8g*

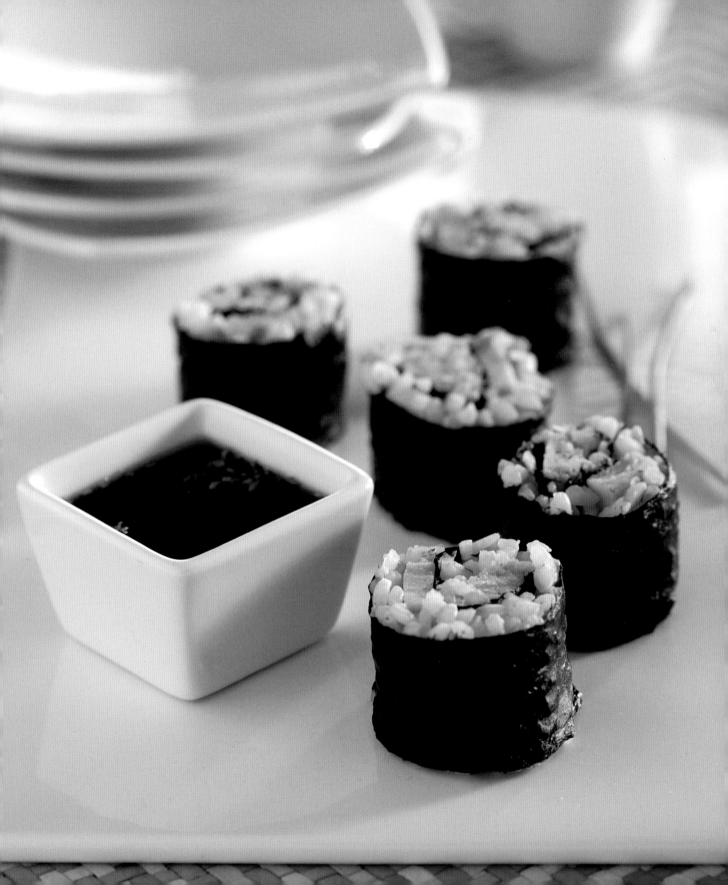

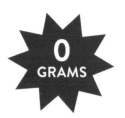

0 GRAMS

MINT-GREEN TEA COOLERS

makes 2 servings

2   bags green tea

4   thin slices fresh ginger
    (about 1 inch)

7   or 8 large fresh mint leaves,
    roughly torn

2   cups boiling water

2   cups crushed ice

1. Place tea bags, ginger and mint leaves in teapot or 2-cup heatproof measuring cup. Add boiling water; steep 4 minutes. Remove tea bags, ginger and mint leaves; discard. Cool tea to room temperature.

2. Pour 1 cup crushed ice into each of two tall glasses. Divide tea between glasses.

SERVING SUGGESTION: Squeeze a lime wedge (about ⅛ of a lime) into each cooler before serving.

nutritionals

Serving Size: *½ of recipe*, Calories: *15*, Total Fat: *0g*, Saturated Fat: *0g*, Cholesterol: *0mg*, Sodium: *0mg*, Carbohydrate: *3g*, Dietary Fiber: *1g*, Sugar: *0g*, Protein: *0g*

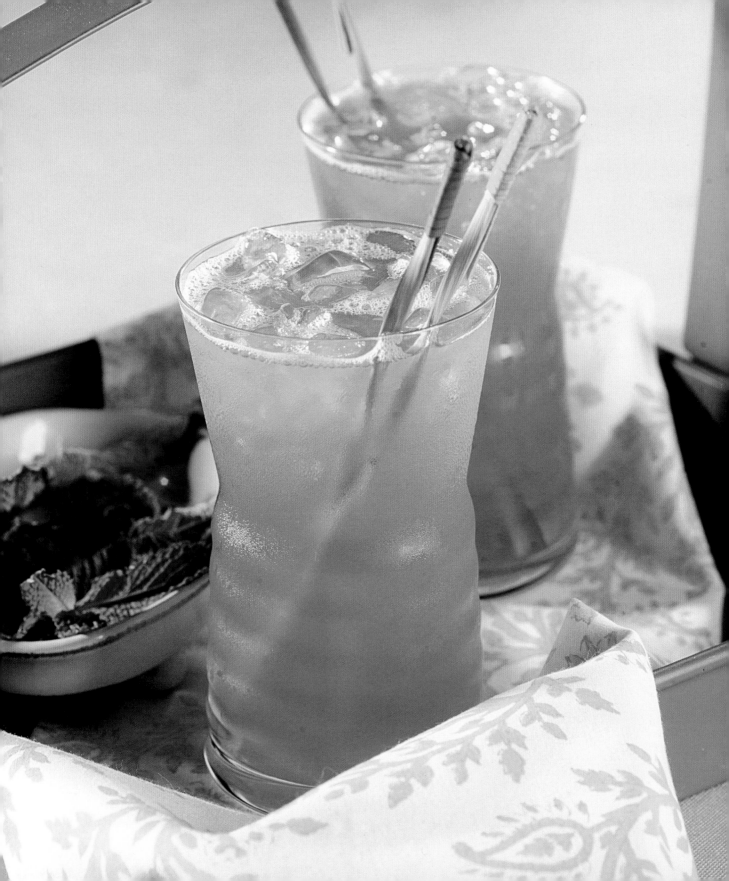

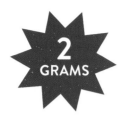

2 GRAMS

HERBED STUFFED TOMATOES

makes 5 servings

15 cherry tomatoes

½ cup (2%) cottage cheese

1 tablespoon thinly sliced
   green onion

1 teaspoon chopped fresh
   chervil *or* ¼ teaspoon
   dried chervil

½ teaspoon snipped fresh dill
   or ⅛ teaspoon dried dill
   weed

⅛ teaspoon lemon-pepper
   seasoning

1. Cut thin slice off bottom of each tomato. Scoop out pulp with small spoon; discard pulp. Invert tomatoes onto paper towels to drain.

2. Stir cottage cheese, green onion, chervil, dill and lemon-pepper seasoning in small bowl until just combined. Spoon evenly into tomatoes. Serve immediately or cover and refrigerate up to 8 hours.

nutritionals

Serving Size: *3 stuffed tomatoes*, Calories: *30*, Total Fat: *1g*, Saturated Fat: *0g*, Cholesterol: *5mg*, Sodium: *80mg*, Carbohydrate: *3g*, Dietary Fiber: *1g*, Sugar: *2g*, Protein: *3g*

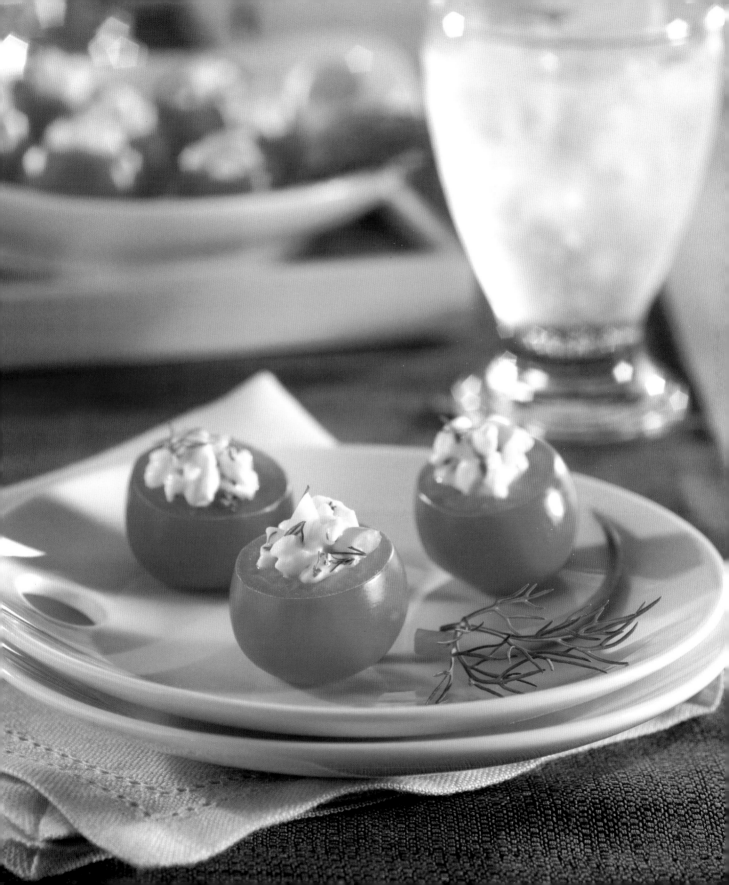

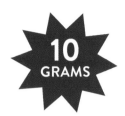

10 GRAMS

FRUIT KABOBS WITH RASPBERRY YOGURT DIP

makes 6 servings

½ cup plain nonfat yogurt

2 tablespoons no-sugar-added raspberry fruit spread

1 pint fresh strawberries

2 cups cubed honeydew melon (1-inch cubes)

2 cups cubed cantaloupe (1-inch cubes)

1 can (8 ounces) pineapple chunks in juice, drained

1. Stir yogurt and fruit spread in small bowl until well blended.

2. Thread fruit alternately onto six 12-inch skewers. Serve with yogurt dip.

nutritionals

Serving Size: *½ kabob with 1 tablespoon dip*, Calories: *50*, Total Fat: *0g*, Saturated Fat: *0g*, Cholesterol: *0mg*, Sodium: *20mg*, Carbohydrate: *12g*, Dietary Fiber: *1g*, Sugar: *10g*, Protein: *1g*

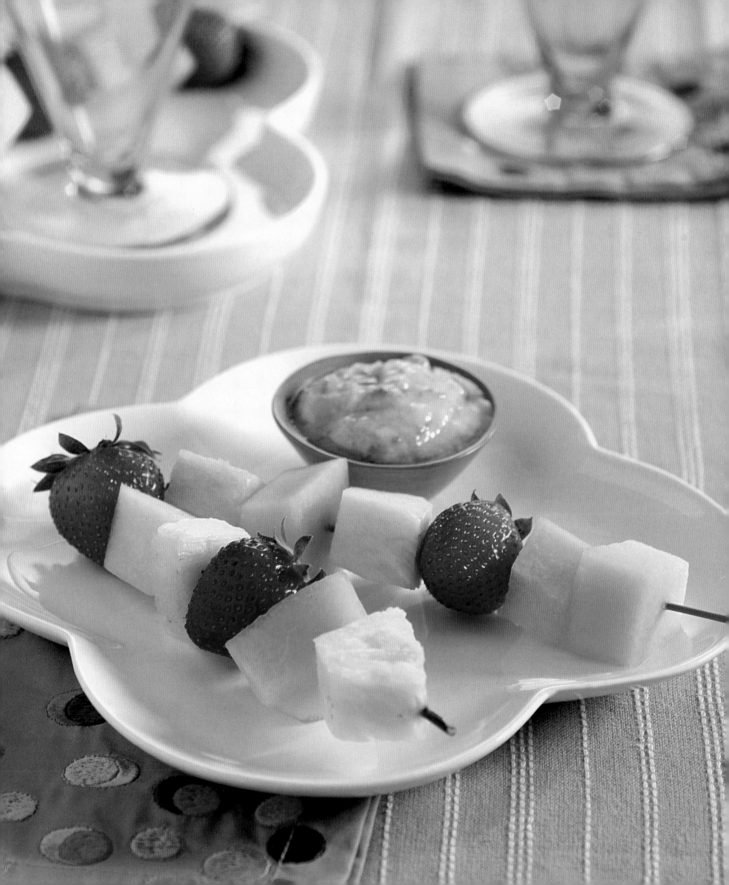

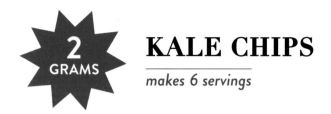

2 GRAMS

KALE CHIPS

makes 6 servings

1 large bunch kale (about
    1 pound)
1 to 2 tablespoons olive oil
1 teaspoon garlic salt or other
    seasoned salt

1. Preheat oven to 350°F. Line baking sheets with parchment paper.

2. Wash kale and pat dry with paper towels. Remove center ribs and stems; discard. Cut leaves into 2- to 3-inch-wide pieces.

3. Combine leaves, oil and garlic salt in large bowl; toss to coat. Spread onto prepared baking sheets.

4. Bake 10 to 15 minutes or until edges are lightly browned and leaves are crisp.* Cool completely on baking sheets.

   If the leaves are lightly browned but not crisp, turn oven off and let chips stand in oven until crisp, about 10 minutes. Do not keep the oven on as the chips will burn easily.

---

nutritionals

Serving Size: *⅙ of recipe*, Calories: *60*, Total Fat: *3g*, Saturated Fat: *0g*, Cholesterol: *0mg*, Sodium: *230mg*, Carbohydrate: *7g*, Dietary Fiber: *3g*, Sugar: *2g*, Protein: *3g*

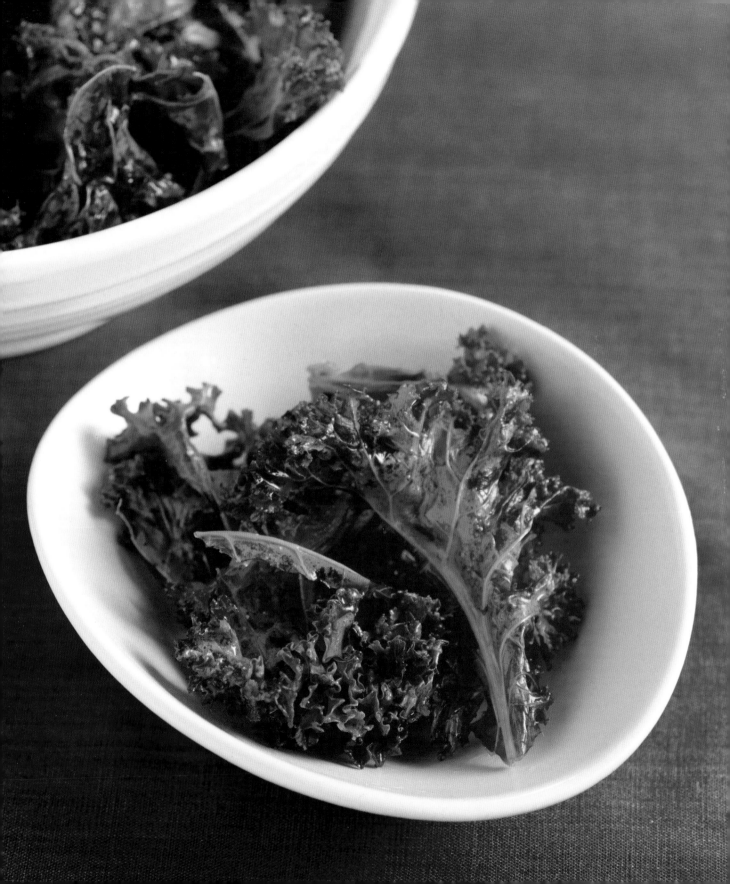

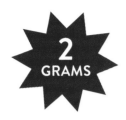

2 GRAMS

SPICY ROASTED CHICKPEAS

makes 4 servings

1 can (about 15 ounces) chickpeas, rinsed and drained

3 tablespoons olive oil

½ teaspoon salt

½ teaspoon black pepper

¾ to 1 tablespoon chili powder

⅛ to ¼ teaspoon ground red pepper

1 lime, cut into wedges

1. Preheat oven to 400°F.

2. Combine chickpeas, oil, salt and black pepper in large bowl; toss to coat. Spread in single layer on 15×10-inch jelly-roll pan.

3. Bake 15 minutes or until chickpeas begin to brown, shaking pan twice.

4. Sprinkle with chili powder and red pepper. Bake 5 minutes or until dark golden-red. Serve with lime wedges.

nutritionals

Serving Size: *½ cup*, Calories: *120*, Total Fat: *5g*, Saturated Fat: *0g*, Cholesterol: *0mg*, Sodium: *540mg*, Carbohydrate: *16g*, Dietary Fiber: *4g*, Sugar: *2g*, Protein: *4g*

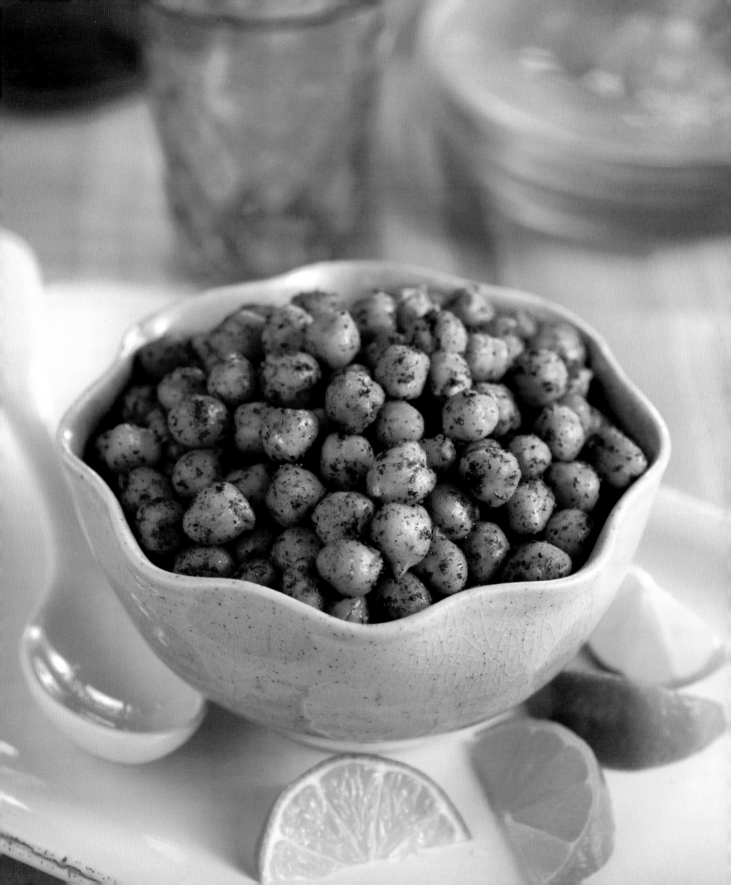

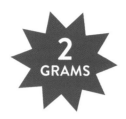
2 GRAMS

FROSTY RASPBERRY LEMON TEA

makes 2 servings

1½ cups ice

1 cup brewed lemon-flavored herbal tea, at room temperature

1 cup water

½ cup frozen unsweetened raspberries

1. Combine ice, tea, water and raspberries in blender or food processor; blend until smooth, pulsing to break up ice.

2. Pour into two glasses. Serve immediately.

nutritionals

Serving Size: *½ of recipe*, Calories: *20*, Total Fat: *0g*, Saturated Fat: *0g*, Cholesterol: *0mg*, Sodium: *0mg*, Carbohydrate: *5g*, Dietary Fiber: *2g*, Sugar: *2g*, Protein: *0g*

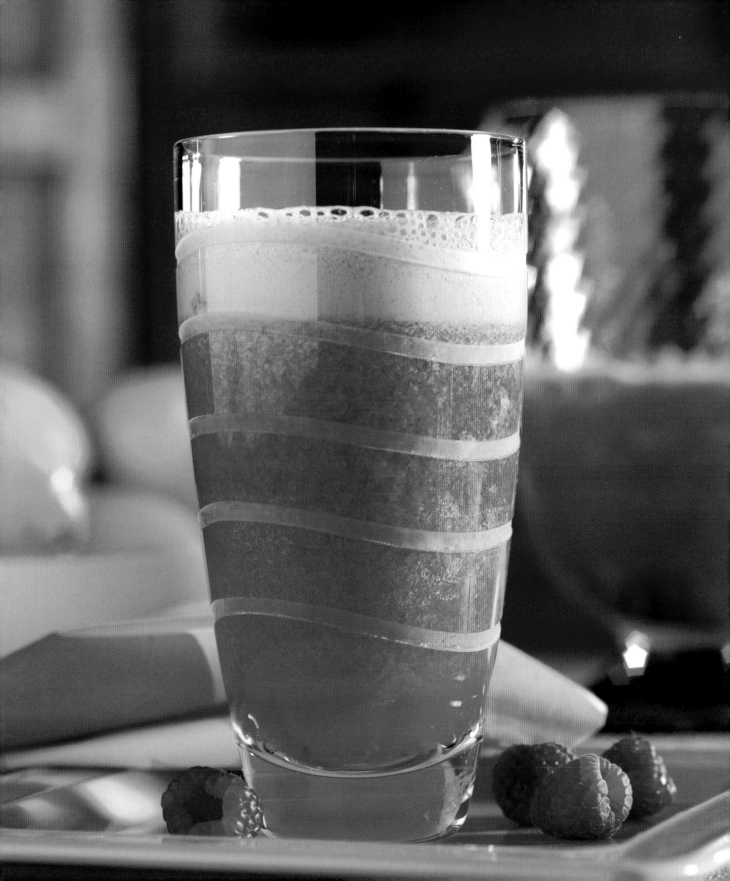

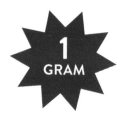

1 GRAM

MEDITERRANEAN-STYLE DEVILED EGGS

makes 6 servings

¼ cup finely diced cucumber

¼ cup finely diced tomato

2 teaspoons fresh lemon juice

⅛ teaspoon salt

6 hard-cooked eggs, peeled and sliced in half lengthwise

⅓ cup roasted garlic or any flavor hummus

Chopped fresh parsley (optional)

1. Combine cucumber, tomato, lemon juice and salt in small bowl; gently mix.

2. Remove yolks from eggs; discard. Spoon 1 heaping teaspoon hummus into each egg half. Top with ½ teaspoon cucumber-tomato mixture and parsley, if desired. Serve immediately.

---

nutritionals

Serving Size: *2 halves*, Calories: *100*, Total Fat: *7g*, Saturated Fat: *2g*, Cholesterol: *185mg*, Sodium: *160mg*, Carbohydrate: *3g*, Dietary Fiber: *0g*, Sugar: *1g*, Protein: *7g*

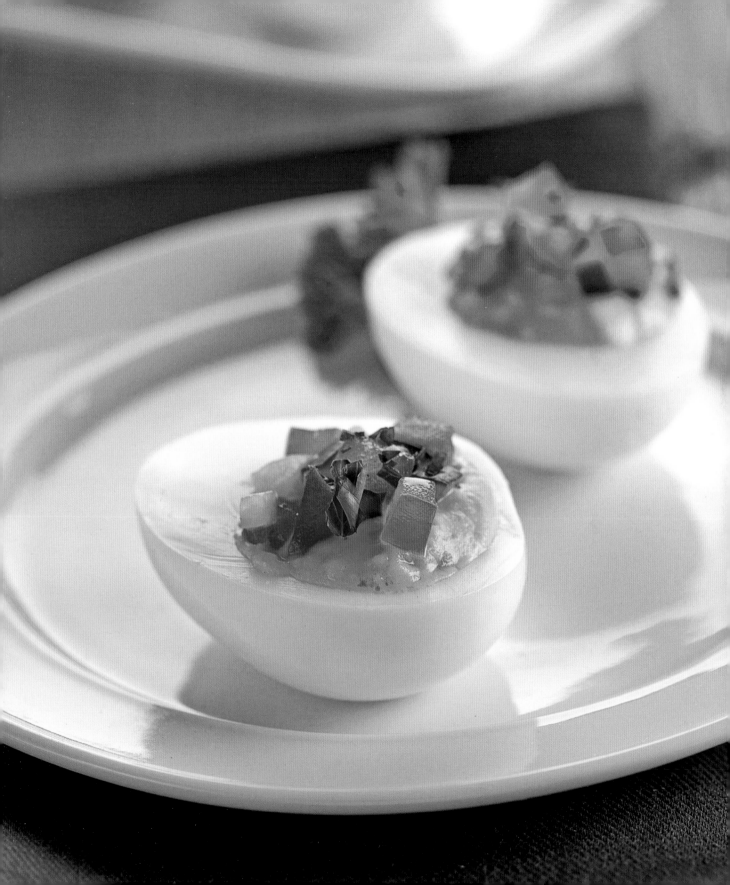

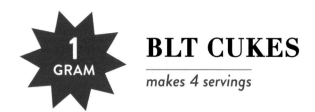

1 GRAM

BLT CUKES

makes 4 servings

½ cup finely chopped lettuce

½ cup finely chopped baby spinach

3 slices bacon, crisp-cooked and crumbled

¼ cup finely diced tomato

1 tablespoon plus 1½ teaspoons mayonnaise

¼ teaspoon black pepper

⅛ teaspoon salt

1 large cucumber

Minced fresh parsley or green onion (optional)

1. Combine lettuce, spinach, bacon, tomato, mayonnaise, pepper and salt in medium bowl; mix well.

2. Peel cucumber; trim off ends and cut in half lengthwise. Use spoon to scoop out seeds; discard seeds.

3. Divide bacon mixture between cucumber halves, mounding in center. Garnish with parsley. Cut each half into eight 2-inch pieces.

TIP: Make these snacks when cucumbers are plentiful and large enough to easily hollow out with a spoon. These snacks can be made, covered and refrigerated up to 12 hours ahead of time.

nutritionals

Serving Size: *4 pieces*, Calories: *70*, Total Fat: *5g*, Saturated Fat: *1g*, Cholesterol: *0mg*, Sodium: *200mg*, Carbohydrate: *2g*, Dietary Fiber: *1g*, Sugar: *1g*, Protein: *3g*

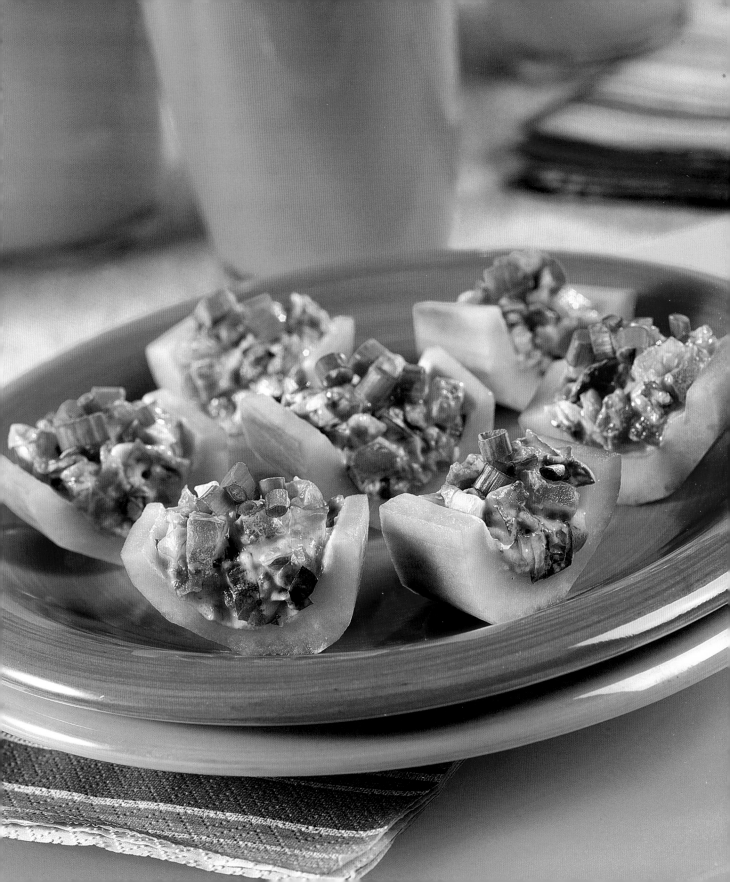

INDEX

METRIC CONVERSION CHART

VOLUME
MEASUREMENTS (dry)

$\frac{1}{8}$ teaspoon = 0.5 mL
$\frac{1}{4}$ teaspoon = 1 mL
$\frac{1}{2}$ teaspoon = 2 mL
$\frac{3}{4}$ teaspoon = 4 mL
1 teaspoon = 5 mL
1 tablespoon = 15 mL
2 tablespoons = 30 mL
$\frac{1}{4}$ cup = 60 mL
$\frac{1}{3}$ cup = 75 mL
$\frac{1}{2}$ cup = 125 mL
$\frac{2}{3}$ cup = 150 mL
$\frac{3}{4}$ cup = 175 mL
1 cup = 250 mL
2 cups = 1 pint = 500 mL
3 cups = 750 mL
4 cups = 1 quart = 1 L

VOLUME MEASUREMENTS (fluid)

1 fluid ounce (2 tablespoons) = 30 mL
4 fluid ounces ($\frac{1}{2}$ cup) = 125 mL
8 fluid ounces (1 cup) = 250 mL
12 fluid ounces (1$\frac{1}{2}$ cups) = 375 mL
16 fluid ounces (2 cups) = 500 mL

WEIGHTS (mass)

$\frac{1}{2}$ ounce = 15 g
1 ounce = 30 g
3 ounces = 90 g
4 ounces = 120 g
8 ounces = 225 g
10 ounces = 285 g
12 ounces = 360 g
16 ounces = 1 pound = 450 g

DIMENSIONS

$\frac{1}{16}$ inch = 2 mm
$\frac{1}{8}$ inch = 3 mm
$\frac{1}{4}$ inch = 6 mm
$\frac{1}{2}$ inch = 1.5 cm
$\frac{3}{4}$ inch = 2 cm
1 inch = 2.5 cm

OVEN
TEMPERATURES

250°F = 120°C
275°F = 140°C
300°F = 150°C
325°F = 160°C
350°F = 180°C
375°F = 190°C
400°F = 200°C
425°F = 220°C
450°F = 230°C

BAKING PAN SIZES

Utensil	Size in Inches/Quarts	Metric Volume	Size in Centimeters
Baking or Cake Pan (square or rectangular)	8×8×2	2 L	20×20×5
	9×9×2	2.5 L	23×23×5
	12×8×2	3 L	30×20×5
	13×9×2	3.5 L	33×23×5
Loaf Pan	8×4×3	1.5 L	20×10×7
	9×5×3	2 L	23×13×7
Round Layer Cake Pan	8×1½	1.2 L	20×4
	9×1½	1.5 L	23×4
Pie Plate	8×1¼	750 mL	20×3
	9×1¼	1 L	23×3
Baking Dish or Casserole	1 quart	1 L	—
	1½ quart	1.5 L	—
	2 quart	2 L	—